NUTRITION AND DIET RESEARCH PROGRESS

DIETARY PLANT PRODUCTS AND HUMAN HEALTH: NEW EVIDENCES ABOUT THE EFFECTS ON DEGENERATIVE DISEASES

NUTRITION AND DIET RESEARCH PROGRESS

Additional books in this series can be found on Nova's website under the Series tab.

AGRICULTURE ISSUES AND POLICIES

Additional books in this series can be found on Nova's website under the Series tab.

NUTRITION AND DIET RESEARCH PROGRESS

DIETARY PLANT PRODUCTS AND HUMAN HEALTH: NEW EVIDENCES ABOUT THE EFFECTS ON DEGENERATIVE DISEASES

MAURO SERAFINI
AND
CRISTIANA MIGLIO

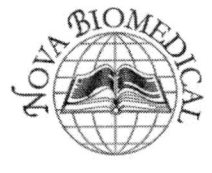

Nova Science Publishers, Inc.
New York

Copyright © 2011 by Nova Science Publishers, Inc.

All rights reserved. No part of this book may be reproduced, stored in a retrieval system or transmitted in any form or by any means: electronic, electrostatic, magnetic, tape, mechanical photocopying, recording or otherwise without the written permission of the Publisher.

For permission to use material from this book please contact us:
Telephone 631-231-7269; Fax 631-231-8175
Web Site: http://www.novapublishers.com

NOTICE TO THE READER

The Publisher has taken reasonable care in the preparation of this book, but makes no expressed or implied warranty of any kind and assumes no responsibility for any errors or omissions. No liability is assumed for incidental or consequential damages in connection with or arising out of information contained in this book. The Publisher shall not be liable for any special, consequential, or exemplary damages resulting, in whole or in part, from the readers' use of, or reliance upon, this material. Any parts of this book based on government reports are so indicated and copyright is claimed for those parts to the extent applicable to compilations of such works.

Independent verification should be sought for any data, advice or recommendations contained in this book. In addition, no responsibility is assumed by the publisher for any injury and/or damage to persons or property arising from any methods, products, instructions, ideas or otherwise contained in this publication.

This publication is designed to provide accurate and authoritative information with regard to the subject matter covered herein. It is sold with the clear understanding that the Publisher is not engaged in rendering legal or any other professional services. If legal or any other expert assistance is required, the services of a competent person should be sought. FROM A DECLARATION OF PARTICIPANTS JOINTLY ADOPTED BY A COMMITTEE OF THE AMERICAN BAR ASSOCIATION AND A COMMITTEE OF PUBLISHERS.

Additional color graphics may be available in the e-book version of this book.

Library of Congress Cataloging-in-Publication Data

Serafini, Mauro.
  Dietary plant products and human health : new evidences about the effects on degenerative diseases / authors: Mauro Serafini and Cristiana Miglio.
     p. cm.
    Includes index.
    ISBN 978-1-61209-672-8 (softcover)
   1. Vegetables--Therapeutic use. 2. Fruit--Therapeutic use. 3. Diet therapy. I. Miglio, Cristiana. II. Title.
    RM236.S47 2011
    615.8'54--dc22
                                     2011001421

Published by Nova Science Publishers, Inc. ✝ New York

Contents

Preface		**vii**
Chapter I	Introduction	**1**
Chapter II	Epidemiological Evidence on the Role of Fruit and Vegetable in the Protection of Chronic Diseases	**5**
Chapter III	Health Effects of Fruit and Vegetables: Which Mechanism of Action?	**23**
Chapter IV	Antioxidant Activity	**25**
Chapter V	Endocrine Regulation	**33**
Chapter VI	Other Mechanisms	**35**
Chapter VII	Conclusions	**39**
References		**41**
Index		**57**

Preface

Plant-based foods such as fruit and vegetables, nuts, natural vegetable oils, and whole grains are an important component of traditional diets in Mediterranean regions. A large and consistent body of scientific evidence has provided solid evidences about the role of plant food-based diet as a whole, in the prevention of degenerative diseases.Despite evidenceshave been produced on the protective role of the so-called phytochemicals, a wide variety of bioactive non-nutrient compounds present in the vegetable kingdom, it is still unclear which components of the diet are protective and what are their mechanisms of actions. To further complicate the picture, very latest findings, suggest the lack of a causal effect between fruit and vegetable consumption and cancer prevention, highlighting the need for future research. The first part of this chapter intends to provide an overview of the evidence describing the health-promoting benefits of the consumption of plant food-based diets. The second part of this chapter will illustrate the possible mechanisms through which the protection is carried out.

Chapter I

Introduction

Throughout human history, societies have developed many ways to combine the foods that are available as a result of geography, climate, trade or cultural preferences into their particular dietary patterns or cuisines. Plant-based foods are an important component of traditional diets in Mediterranean regions (Ferro-Luzzi&Sette 1989). The exact definition of what the Mediterranean diet consists of is somewhat controversial, particularly as far as the amount of total fat is concerned, but common features are the centrality of cereals, legumes, fruit and vegetables, the moderate consumption of fish, milk and dairy products, the low consumption of meat and meat products, the use of extra-virgin olive oil as main dressing, as well as the moderate intake of red wine. This translates into high intake of carbohydrates, particularly starch, low intake of saturated fatty acids, high monounsaturated/saturated fatty acid ratio, high vegetal to animal protein ratio, high intake of potassium, vitamins (except maybe vitamin D), marginal intake of iron and zinc, and high intake of bioactive compounds (Ferro-Luzzi & Branca 1995).

Biochemical, clinical and epidemiological research during the past 20 years has provided a solid foundation for the health benefits of the Mediterranean diet, which is consistent with lower incidence of Cardio-vascular Disease (CVD), several types of cancers and Parkinson's and Alzheimer's diseases (Reddy & Katan 2004; Martínez-González and Sánchez-Villegas 2004, Sofi et al. 2008, Mente et al. 2009), as well as reduction in overall mortality (Sofi et al. 2008, Trichopoulou et al. 2009). The relative importance of single components of the Mediterranean diet as predictor of lower mortality has not been deeply understood yet, but there is a general consensus from the available evidence, that higher intake of fruit and vegetables is beneficial for human health. For this reason, it is now established by world-round public health bodies that high consumption of fruit and vegetables is beneficial and many public campaigns are conducted in order to increase public awareness.

Since their first appearance in the late 1950s (Keys & Keys 1959) dietary guidelines for disease prevention have recommended people to eat more fruits and vegetables.In 1982 the National Academy of Sciences issued guidelines emphasizing the importance of fruit and vegetables in the diet. The Food Guide Pyramid encourages up to 9 servings of fruit and vegetables daily for general good health (USDA 1992). In 1991, the 5-A-Day Program for Better Health was initiated by the National Cancer Institute and the Produce for Better Health Foundation. After the American initiative, the 5 a day program was adopted by several European countries. The USDA and the American Health Association (USDA 1995; AHA 1996) reports recommend consuming 5 or more servings of fruit and vegetables daily, in order to reduce the risk of both cancer and heart disease and to promote an adequate vitamin intake. In March 2007, the 5 A Day program became the National Fruit and Vegetable Program and a new public health initiative, the so called "Fruits & Veggies—More Matters", was launched, in order to reflect the new dietary guidelines, which, both in USA and in Europe, recommend more than 5 servings of fruits and vegetables a day (USDA 2005; EUFIC 2009).

However, despite the large consensus on benefits of diets rich in plant foods, several points are still obscure and there is a large uncertainty as to which components of plant-based foods are protective and what are their mechanisms of action. Epidemiological and experimental evidence is available on previously unrecognized properties of the so-called phytochemicals present in fruit and vegetables (Knekt et al. 1996; Go et al. 2003; Surh YJ. 2003). Phytochemicals are bioactive non-nutrient compounds which are widely present in plant food with different chemical structures and modality of action. In general, the phytochemicals function by attracting beneficial organisms and repelling harmful organisms; they also serve as photoprotectants, and respond to environmental changes (Lampe 2003). Extensive studies of phytochemicals in cell-culture and in animal models have provided a wealth of information on the different modality of action of these molecules (Lampe 2003). Different phytochemicals have been shown to possess antioxidant, antimicrobial, antiviral anti-inflammatory activities, to modulate detoxification enzymes, stimulate immune function, decrease platelet aggregation, modulate hormone metabolism and affect cholesterol metabolism (Lampe 1999). However, despite the increasing evidence suggesting the crucial role played by phytochemicals, the identification of single active compounds is far from been reached.

The first part of this chapter intends to provide an overview of the human studies supporting the health-promoting benefits of the consumption of fruit and vegetables. The second part of this chapter will illustrate the possible mechanisms through which the protection action is carried out.

Chapter II

Epidemiological Evidence on the Role of Fruit and Vegetable in the Protection of Chronic Diseases

2.1. Cancer

Carcinogenesis is a complex multi-step process that can be regarded as a disease of cells, characterized by an excess of cells beyond the number needed for normal function of the body organ affected (Halliwell&Gutteridge 1989). The first step of carcinogenesis is initiation: a series of events whereby a carcinogen induces mutation in the cell resulting in transformed or initiated cells. This mutation is either present in the cells or, more often, induced by environmental factors (i.e. ionizing radiation). Food may provide carcinogenic contaminants (xenobiotics) or be a mutagen itself, after some nutrients are transformed. The next step, promotion, is the clonal proliferation of mutated cells that occurs as the result of genetic alterations and epigenetic modulations and will achieve tumor growth. This step involves alterations in gene expression and cell proliferation which transform the cells. The last stage of the cancer process, the invasion step, involves the increased growth and expansion of a population of initiated and promoted cancer cells to an invasive tumor mass, often accompanied by an abnormal complement of genetic material.

Reactive Oxygen Nitrogen Species (RONS) and oxidative stress are thought to be involved into tumorigenesis at different levels. Oxidative damage to DNA, leading to DNA single or double strand breaks and DNA cross linking, as well as to chromosomal aberrations, such as breakage or rearrangement, is the most commonly offered explanation, demonstrated by both *in vitro* and *in vivo* studies (Halliwell 2007). The modifications of DNA bases might result in point mutations, deletions, or gene amplification, representing early-stage steps for carcinogenesis (Halliwell and Gutteridge 1989). However, recent findings that, in some situations, cancer rates do not increase despite highly elevated levels of oxidized DNA bases (Nakabeppu et al. 2004), suggest that oxidative DNA damage may be necessary, but not sufficient, for cancer development and other mechanisms of action by RONS must be involved, including deactivation of detoxifying enzymes responsible for the scavenging of potent carcinogens, their interaction with the tumor suppressor protein p53 and their involvement in chronic inflammation (Halliwell 2007).

Thirty years ago, a landmark study by Doll &Peto concluded that 75–80% of cancers diagnosed in the United States in 1970 might theoretically have been prevented by altering environmental factors such as smoking, alcohol consumption and diet (Doll & Peto 1981) and Steinmeitz & Potter estimated that up to 70% of all cancer is attributable to diet (Steinmeitz & Potter 1996).

With respect to plant foods, fruit and vegetable, as foods rich in bioactive molecules has been subject of intensive investigations for their potential ability to prevent incidence of cancer. The first and most comprehensive review of epidemiologic data was produced by Block et al. in 1992. In this paper, approximately 200 studies were examined, investigating the relationship between fruit and vegetable intake and cancer of the lung, colon, breast, cervix, esophagus, oral cavity, stomach, bladder, pancreas and ovary. The authors showed a statistically significant protective effect of fruit and vegetable consumption in 128 out of 156 dietary studies. For many cancer sites, subjects with a lower intake of fruit and vegetables showed a risk twice as high as people with the highest intake, even after adjustment for potential confounders (age, sex, energy etc). Both fruit and vegetable consumption resulted to be protective against cancers at different sites, including lung (24 out of 25 studies), pancreas and stomach (26 out of 30 studies), colon, rectum and bladder (23 out of 38 studies) and cervix, ovary and endometrium (11 out of 13). Moreover, fruits were highly protective in cancers of the esophagus, oral cavity and larynx (28 out of 29 studies).

In the late nineties, both the World Cancer Research Fund with the American Institute for Cancer Research (WCRF-AICR) and the Chief Medical Officer's Committee on Medical Aspects of Food and Nutrition Policy of the

United Kingdom (COMA) produced a report in which an exhaustive collection of worldwide research on food nutrition and cancer was reviewed. A summary of the results from the two reports are outlined in Table 1. In the WCRF report, more than 250 case-control and cohort studies were reviewed (WCRF 1997). Among the different types of cancer, the experts concluded that there was convincing evidence that a high intake of vegetables decreases the risk of cancer at mouth and pharynx, esophagus, lung, stomach, colon and rectum sites.They also stated that vegetable consumption probably decreases the risk of cancer of the larynx, pancreas, breast and bladder and that it may decrease the risk of cancer of the liver, ovary, endometrium, cervix, prostate, thyroid and kidney (Table 1). Fruit consumption was also associated with a decrease of the risk of the aforementioned types of cancer with the exception of the liver, prostate, kidney, colon and rectum, for which the existing evidence was considered limited or inconsistent. Similar conclusions were drawn in the report commissioned by the COMA (1998), as described in Table 1.Both reports agreed on the protective effect of fruit and vegetables against cancer of the bladder, breast, colon, rectum and larynx. Nonetheless, for other site-specific cancers there is some disagreement between the two panels, mainly due to the different criteria used to classify the strength of evidence. Based on these evidences, the WCRF-AICR report estimated that "diets high in fruit and vegetables could prevent at least 20% of all cancer incidences and set a target daily consumption of 400 up to 800 g of different varieties of fruit and vegetables (WCRF 1997). In keeping with the WCRF-AICR recommendations, the COMA (1998) report suggested increasing intakes of a wide variety of fruit and vegetables, although without quantifying an optimum level of intake, but merely stating that any increase would be expected to be beneficial.

In following years, further findings coming out from an extensive investigation in this field, led to somehow different conclusions. The results available at the time of the two reports (WCRF-AICR and COMA) derived mainly from case-control studies, in which dietary information from people with cancer (cases) were compared with information from healthy people (controls).

Table 1. Summary of main conclusion from the review of epidemiologic evidences on the effect of fruit and vegetable consumption against cancer (Source: WCRF 1997, 2007 and COMA 1998) [1]

Cancer site	COMA 1998[2]	WCRF-AICR 1997[2]	WCRF-AICR 2007[2]
Bladder	2	2	4
Breast	2 for vegetables 3 for fruits	2	4 (3 only for carrots)
Cervix	1, limited data	3	4
Colon and rectum	1	1	3
Endometrium	4	3	4 for fruit 3 for vegetable
Esophagus	2 for vegetables 5 for fruit	1 for vegetables 4 for fruit	2
Kidney	Not included	3	4
Larynx	2, limited data	2	Not included
Liver	Not included	2	4 for vegetables 3 for fruits
Lung	2 for fruit, 3 for vegetables	1	3 for vegetable 2 for fruit
Mouth, pharynx and larynx	5 for vegetables, larynx excluded 3 for fruit, larynx excluded	1, larynx excluded	2
Nasopharynx	Not included	Not included	3
Ovary	4	3	4 for vegetable 3 for fruit
Pancreas	1, limited data	2	4 for vegetable 3 for fruits
Prostate	2	3	4
Stomach	2	1	2
Skyn	Not included	Not included	4

[1] WCRF-AICR, World Cancer Research Fund-American Institute for Cancer Research; COMA, Chief Medical Officer's Committee on Medical Aspects of Food and Nutrition Policy of the United Kingdom.

[2] Strength of evidences for WCRF 1997: convincing = 1, probable = 2, possible = 3 and limited = 4; for WCRF 2007: convincing = 1, probable = 2 and limited-suggestive = 3, limited-no conclusion = 4; and for COMA: strongly consistent = 1, moderately consistent = 2, weakly consistent = 3, insufficient = 4, inconsistent = 5.

These kinds of studies are susceptible to recall biases, as cases may have changed diet during the study period. More recent results coming from large prospective cohort studies, where dietary intakes are evaluated at recruitment and then people are followed up for cancer incidence, and from few available intervention trials, in which volunteers are asked to follow specific dietary patterns or to supplement their habitual diet, do not support the view that fruit and vegetables have a strong protective effect in the prevention of certain site-specific types of cancer, suggesting that some previous observations were ambiguous (Timothy et al. 2002).

Riboli and Norat (2003) conducted a meta-analysis of both case-control and cohort studies, published between 1973 and 2001. In this study, although case-control studies overall supported a significant reduction in the risks of cancers of the esophagus, lung, stomach, and colorectum associated with both fruit and vegetables, of breast cancer associated only with vegetables, and of bladder cancer associated only with fruit, the overall relative risk estimates from cohort studies suggested a protective effect of both fruit and vegetables for most cancer sites considered, but the risk reduction resulted to be significant only for cancers of the lung and bladder and only for fruit (Riboli and Norat 2003). In a meta-analyses on eight prospective cohort studies published between 1989 and 1999, including 7,377 incident invasive breast cancer cases occurring among 351,825 women whose diet was analyzed at baseline, no association was found between fruit and vegetable and breast cancer risk (Smith-Warner et al. 2001). The Health Professionals Follow up study, a prospective cohort study, initiated in 1986 and involving 51,529 American men aged 40–75 years, found no relation for dietary intake of potassium, sodium, calcium, magnesium, phosphorus, iron, or water-soluble vitamins and bladder cancer risk. (Michaud et al. 2000). Regarding lung cancer, three prospective studies described fruit and vegetable protective effects, but without reaching any statistical significance (Feskanich et al. 2000; Voorrips et al. 2000; Jansen et al. 2001).

Based on these new findings, in 2003, the International Agency for Research on Cancer (IARC) classified the evidences for a protective role of fruit and vegetables on cancer as "limited" (IARC 2003). In 2007, the WCRF produced a new report, in which the experts downgraded the strength of the evidence for all the cancer sites, for which the health effect has been previously judged "convincing" or "probable". The new results are also reported in Table 1. The matrices used in 2007 differed from those used in 1997, in some respects: the categories of "possible" and "insufficient" were substituted by the categories of "limited-suggestive" and "limited no conclusion", whereas the judgments of "convincing" and "probable" remained common to both reports (WCRF 2007). The 2007 report suggest a probable protective role for fruit and vegetables against cancers of the esophagus, mouth, pharynx and larynx, stomach, and of lung for fruit only. A "suggestive" protection was indicated for colon and rectum, nose-pharynx, for pancreas and liver in case of fruits and for ovary, endometrium and lung in case of vegetables. No associations with specific cancer sites were found to be "convincing" (WCRF 2007).

A further support to the notion of a modest cancer preventive effect of high intake of fruits and vegetables came from recent prospective analyses of the National Institutes of Health–AARP Diet and Health cohort, in the United States (George et al. 2009) and the European Prospective Investigation into Cancer and Nutrition cohort (EPIC), in Europe (Boffetta et al. 2010). In the first study the authors sought to investigate the association of fruit and vegetable intake and incidence of cancer of the leading sites, as well as total cancers, in a cohort of288,109 men and 195,229 women, aged more than 50 years (George et al. 2009). The second study investigated the relationship between high fruit and vegetable intake and cancer for all causes, in a total of 142,605 men and 335,873 women from 10 different European countries (Boffetta et al. 2010). Vegetable intake was not associated with risk neither of total cancer nor for specific cancer sites among women, but was associated with a significant decrease in risk in men. However, this significant finding among men was no longer evident when the authors limited the analysis to men who never smoked (George et al. 2009). On the other hand,Boffetta et al. found only a weak inverse association between higher intakes of fruit and vegetable and overall cancer risk.

High intakes of fruit and vegetables are usually associated with other healthy lifestyle factors, including lower intake of alcohol, never or short duration-smokingand higher level of physical activity, which may also contribute to lower cancer incidence (Boffetta et al. 2010). At epidemiological level, these confounding variables may have masked the results, leading to an overestimation of fruit and vegetables protection against cancer.

Although fruit and vegetable intake is still encouraged by national authorities for many reasons related to overall health, energy balance and nutritional requirements, the wide body of scientific evidence produced in the last decade, partially hampered the enthusiasm aboutthe preventive effect of fruit and vegetables against cancer development, suggesting more caution in the interpretation of the scientific findings.

2.2. Cardiovascular Diseases (CVD)

Cardiovascular diseases are the class of diseases that involve the blood vessels (arteries and veins). While the term technically refers to any disease that affects the cardiovascular system, it is usually used to refer to those related to atherosclerosis, including coronary heart diseases (CHD) and stroke.

In Western populations half of the mortality is due to diseases of the cardiovascular system in which the main pathophysiological factor is atherosclerosis. Atherogenesis is a chronic inflammatory process that involves a complex interplay between circulating cellular and blood elements within the cells of the artery wall (Steinberg & Witzum 1990; Ross 1999). This process occurs at a young age in the arteries as accumulation of lipids in the subintimal area, known as fatty streaks (Stary et al. 1995). Fatty streaks consist of sub-endothelial aggregates of lipid-laden foam cells, predominantly macrophages. Fatty streaks may regress, alternatively they may progress to fibrous plaques, which represent the characteristic lesions of advancing atherosclerosis. The fibrous plaque comprises mainly smooth muscle cells and is the product of cytokines and growth factors. The fibrous plaques may undergo calcification, necrosis, hemorrhage, ulceration or thrombosis to form a complex lesion that is most commonly associated with clinical atherosclerosis (Iuliano 2001).

Clinical, genetic and epidemiological studies demonstrate that oxidative stress, and particularly oxidation of LDL, is a risk factor and plays a significant pathogenic role for atherosclerotic diseases (Parthasarathy et al. 1998; Diplock et al. 1998; Parthasarathy et al. 1999; Witzum & Steinberg 2001, Bruckdorfer 2008). LDL oxidation is due to a lipid peroxidation reaction initiated by free radical species. Research studies on the lipid and protein parts of oxidized LDL have demonstrated that oxidative modifications of both contribute to the pro-atherogenic properties of oxidized LDL. Several biochemical mechanisms underlying this effect have been discussed (Witzum& Steinberg 2001, Bruckdorfer 2008). These include the formation of foam cells on the uptake of oxidized LDL via the scavenger receptor by macrophages resident in the sub-endothelial area, release of cytotoxic lipid peroxidation products from oxidized LDL, or chemo attractant properties of the oxidized lipoproteins.

First evidences of a dietary role of fruit and vegetables in CVD prevention came from epidemiologic investigations. In 1997, Ness and Powles reviewed 36 among ecological, case-control and cohort studies, published in the years from 1966 to 1995, investigating the association between the consumption of fruit and vegetables or surrogate nutrients, and CHD, stroke and total circulatory diseases. Nine of 10 ecological, 2 of 3 case-control and 6 of 16 cohort studies found a significant protective association with CHD; 3 of 5 ecological, none (of 1) case-control and 6 of 8 cohort studies found a significant protective association with stroke and 1 of 2 cohort studies reported a significant protective association with total circulatory diseases (Ness &Powles1997). A stronger evidence of the benefit of increasing fruit and vegetable intake as a means to prevent CVD came from Van't Veer et al. (2000). The authors performed a meta-analysis using results from 14 observational epidemiologic studies (3 case-control and 11 prospective studies) published up to 1998. In this study, they estimated that a 16% reduction of cardiovascular deaths could be achieved by increasing the average fruit and vegetable intake by 150 g/day. In the same years, intervention studies had also advanced, in relation to the link between diet and CVD, further supporting the epidemiological evidence. Main emphasis has been focused on the potential preventive role of individual components of fruit and vegetables. The results allowed the researchers to make the assumption that higher intakes of dietary fibre, folate or antioxidants were associated with lower risk of CVD (Rimm et al. 1995; Kushi et al.1996; Knekt et al.1996; Rimm et al. 1996; Ascherio et al. 1998; Law et al.1998).

Based on these evidences, the 2003 expert report, published by the World Health Organisation (WHO) and the Food and Agriculture Organization of the United Nations (FAO), graded the association for consumption of fruits and vegetables and reduced risk of CVD as convincing. As for recommendation, a daily intake of 400-500 g of fresh fruit and vegetables (including berries, green leafy and cruciferous vegetables and legumes) was suggested as the adequate quantity to reduce the risk of CHD, stroke and major CVD risk factors, such as diabetes and hypertension (WHO/FAO 2003). In following years, results from prospective studies further supported this association.

In Table 2 are summarised the results from cohort studies conducted in USA, Europe and Japan and published between 2000 and 2010. Majority of the trials found an inverse relationship between fruit and vegetable consumption and CVD, further supporting previous results. The Women's Health Study, conducted in USA on about 40000 people, showed that, after adjustment for age and other CVD risk factors, reported a significant inverse association between fruit and vegetable intake and CVD risk (RR: 0.68 for extreme quintiles, 95% CI: 0.51-0.92) (Liu et al. 2000). In North America, The Nurses' Health Study and the Health Professionals Follow-up study indicated that, after adjustment for cardiovascular risk factors, people in the highest quintile of fruit and vegetable intake (between 5 and 6 servings/day) had a RR of IHD of 0.80 (95% CI: 0.69-0.93) compared with the lowest quintile (Joshipura et al. 2001). These results were also equivalent to a consistent reduction in CHD for every 1 serving/day increase in the intake of fruit and vegetables, up to 6 servings/day, interestingly showing no apparent further benefit at higher intakes. In 2002, Bazzano and colleagues studied 9,608 adults aged 25–74 years, participating in the first National Health and Nutrition Examination Survey Epidemiologic Follow-up Study. The authors found that consuming 3 or more servings/day of fruit and vegetables compared with less than 1, was associated with a 27% lower stroke incidence and a 27% lower overall CVD mortality, after adjustment for established cardiovascular disease risk factors (Bazzano et al. 2002). Among European studies, in the prospective Kuopio Ischaemic Heart Disease Risk factor (KIHD) study on 1,950 Finnish men aged 42-60 years, cardiovascular mortality resulted to be lower for men with the highest consumption of fruits, berries and vegetables. After adjustment for the major CVD risk factors, the RR for men in the highest quintile was 0.59 (95% CI: 0.33-1.06) compared with men in the lowest quintile (Rissanen et al. 2003). Higher childhood intake of vegetables was associated with lower risk of stroke in 4,028 individuals of the Boyd Orr cohort, in Britain (Ness et al. 2005). The European Prospective Investigation into Cancer and Nutrition (EPIC) study followed 10,449 self-reported diabetics for 9 years. CVD mortality was significantly inversely associated with 80g/day increased intake of vegetables, legumes, and fruit (RR 0.88, 95% CI: 0.81-0.95) (Nöthlings et al. 2008). Finally, in Asia, the Japan Collaborative Cohort study for evaluation of Cancer risk (JACC) reported a significant inverse relationship between vegetable intake and CHD-related deaths in 25,206 men and 34,279 women, from 45 communities in Japan, followed up for 13 years (Nagura et al. 2009). Fruit intake was inversely associated with mortality from total stroke (HR 0.67, 95% CI: 0.55-0.81), total CVD (HR 0.75, 95% CI: 0.66, 0.85) and total mortality (HR 0.86, 95% CI: 0.80-0.92), while vegetable intake was inversely associated only with total CVD (HR 0.88, 95% CI: 0.78-0.99). In support of these findings, two systematic reviews showed that, consuming more than 5 servings/day of fruit and vegetables, bring to a reduction of the risk of CHD (17%) and stroke (26%) (He et al. 2006 and 2007).

Table 2. Prospective studies describing associations between intake of fruit and vegetables and CVD (2000-2010)

Reference	Cohort	Country	Subjects (sex[1])	Follow-up	Association	Outcome[2]
Liu 2000	Women's Health Study	USA	39876 M	6	Inverse, significant	CVD risk
Cox 2000	British	UK	1489 M 1900 F	7	Inverse, not significant Inverse, significant	CVD risk
Joshipura 2001	Nurses' Health Study and Health Professionals'	USA	42148 M 84251 F	14 8	Inverse, significant	IHD risk
Liu 2001	Physicians' Health Study (only vegetable)	USA	15220 M	12	Inverse, significant	CHD risk
Bazzano 2002	National Health and Nutrition Examination Survey	USA	9608 M&F	19	Inverse, significant Inverse, not significant Inverse, not significant Inverse, significant	Stroke incidence Stroke mortality IHD mortality CVD mortality
Rissanen 2003	Kuopio Ischaemic Heart Disease Risk Factor	Finland	2682 M	12.8	Inverse, significant	CVD mortality
Steffen 2003	Atherosclerosis Risk in Communities	USA	15792 M&F	11	Inverse, significant Inverse, significant Inverse, notsignificant	CAD mortality CAD incidence stroke risk
Johnsen 2003	Danish Diet Cancer and Health Study	Denmark	54506 M&F	3.09	Inverse, significant	Stroke risk
Sauvaget 2003	Life Span Study	Japan	40349 M&F	18	Inverse, significant	Stroke risk
Dauchet 2004	Prospective Epidemiological Study of Myocardial Infarction	France, North Ireland	8087 M	5	Inverse, notsignificant	CHD risk

Reference	Cohort	Country	Subjects (sex[1])	Follow-up	Association	Outcome[2]
Genkinger 2004	Odyssey	USA	6151 M&F	13	Inverse, notsignificant	CVD
Ness 2005	Boyd Orr	UK	4028 M&F	37	Inverse, significant No association	Stroke risk CHD mortality
Nakamura 2008	Takayama	Japan	13355 M 15724 F	7.33	No association Inverse, significant	CVDmortality
Nothlings 2008	European Perspective into Cancer and Diabetics	Europe	4806 M 56042 F	9	Inverse, significant	CVD mortality
Takachi 2008	Japan Public Health Center-Based Prospective Study	Japan	77891 M&F	5.9	Inverse, significant only for fruit	CVD risk
Nagura 2009	Japan Collaborative Cohort Study	Japan	25206 M 34279 F	13	Inverse, significant Inverse, significant only for vegetable	Stroke mortality CVD mortality
Dauchet 2010	Prospective Epidemiological Study of Myocardial Infarction	France, North Ireland	8060 M	10	Inverse,significant in smokers	CVD risk

[1]M, male; F, female.
[2]CVD, Cardiovascular Disease; CHD, Coronary Heart Disease; CAD, Coronary Artery Disease; IHD, Ischemic Heart Disease.

Very recently, a systematic review of the available evidence on the causal link between diet and CVD was conducted by Mente et al. (2009) on 7,204 individuals, with a mean age of 58 years and followed-up for 1 to 12 years. When considering prospective cohort studies, the authors identified strong evidence of a protective relationship for higher intakes of vegetables, nuts, and monounsaturated fatty acids and for various dietary patterns, including Mediterranean, prudent, and high-quality diets. On the other hand, in randomized controlled trials, only the Mediterranean dietary pattern resulted to be significantly associated with CHD risk reduction (Mente et al. 2009). However, despite the presence of possible confounders might suggest caution in interpreting positive results (Dauchet et al. 2010), the body of evidence suggest an association between plant food consumption and reduced risk for CVD.

2.3. Osteoporosis

Osteoporosis is defined as the progressive systemic skeletal disease, characterised by low bone mass and micro architectural deterioration of bone tissue with a consequent increase of bone fragility and susceptibility to fracture (Royal College of Physicians 2000). Due to ageing of populations and more accurate methods for diagnosis, osteoporosis has been rapidly spread in the past decades, with a major increase of the incidence in postmenopausal women (Reginster 2006). Although wrong dietary patterns are considered one of the modifiable risk factors for osteoporosis incidence, data regarding the effect of modifying lifestyle habits on fracture risk are still scarce. Initial interest was focused on the role of specific nutrients, such as vitamin C, D, K, calcium, magnesium and potassium, but increasing emphasis is now placed on the diet as a whole.

It was in the late sixties when the first suggestion of a role of a diet rich in fruit and vegetables in the osteoporosis prevention was outlined (Wachmann 1968). Since than, observational, experimental, clinical, and intervention studies have been conducted, supporting a positive link between diet and indexes of bone health, such as the bone mineral density (BMD) at different sites and biochemical markers of bone turnover (McTiernan 2009).

The stronger evidence of a protective role of high consumption of fruit and vegetables on BMD come from observational studies conducted in the past two decades. Table 3 lists 14 human epidemiological studies published between 1990 and 2010. First correlations were documented in the older population. In a cross-sectional study on 994 Scottish women aged 45-49 years, New et al. (1997) found that increasing consumption of fruit and a vegetable, leading to higher intakes of potassium, magnesium, fiber and vitamin C, was significantly correlated to BMD. In 2000, the same authors showed that femoral neck BMD was higher in women who had consumed high amounts of fruit in their childhood, than in women who had consumed medium or low amounts. They also pointed out that magnesium and potassium were associated to higher total bone mass and that magnesium intake accounted for about 12% of the variation in the excretion of bone biomarkers (New et al. 2000). Nutrients assumed through higher intakes of fruit and vegetables were correlated with reduced bone loss in both pre and post-menopausal women in a longitudinal study on 891 Scottish subjects, aged 45–55 years and followed-up for 5–7 years (Macdonald et al. 2004). In the contest of the Framingham Heart Study, a correlation was observed between BMD and potassium and magnesium derived from fruit and vegetable intakes, in men and women older than 75 years (Tucker et al. 1999). The study also investigated the 4-year longitudinal change in BMD and showedin men that, higher fruit and vegetable intake was associated with less decline in BMD at the hip (Tucker et al. 1999). In a cross-sectional study of 670 postmenopausal Chinese women aged 48–63 years, the total intake of fruits and vegetables was significantly associated with greater BMD at the whole body and different sites, also after adjusting for age, years since menopause, body weight and height, dietary energy, protein, calcium and physical activities (Chen et al. 2006).

Overall, these studiesconsistently suggest a positive effect of fruit and vegetable consumption on BMD at different sites in adults. However, results were not so homogenous when studies were conducted on younger people. In a cross-sectional study of 330 children aged 8 years, Jones et al. (2001)found no association between nutrient or food intake and BMD, although a significant positive correlation was detected between urinary potassium and BMD.McGartland et al (2004) reported a higher heel BMD in 12- and 15-years old girls who had a higher fruit intake, but not in boys. However, this association disappeared, when adjustment was made for height, weight, pubertal status, activity level, social class, alcohol, smoking, and use of nutritional supplements. Consumption of 3 or more servings of fruit and vegetables/day resulted in more bone area of the radius and whole body, and in lower urinary calcium, in 56 early pubertal girls, with respect to girls consuming less than 3 servings/day (Tylavsky et al. 2004).

Table 3. Epidemiologic tudies describing associations between intake of fruit and vegetable andBody Mineral Density (BMD)

Reference	Country	Subjects	Significant correlations with BMD
Eaton-Evans 1993	UK	77 women	Vegetables
Michaelsson 1995	Sweden	175 women	Potassium
New 1997	UK	994 women	Fruit and vegetables, Potassium, magnesium, fibre, vitamin C
New 1998	UK	165 women	Fruit and vegetables, Potassium
Tucker 1999	USA	229 men, 349 women	Fruit and vegetables, Potassium, magnesium
New 2000	UK	62 women	Fruit and vegetables, Potassium, magnesium, fiber, vitamin C
Jones 2001	Australia	330 children	Urinary Potassium
Whiting 2002	Canada	57 men	Potassium
Macdonald 2004	UK	891 women	Fruit and vegetables, calcium, vitamin C, magnesium, and potassium
MacGartland 2004	Northern Ireland	324 12-y-old boys 378 12-y-old girls 274 15-y-old boys 369 15-y-old girls	No association Fruit No association Fruit
Tylavsky 2004	USA	56 prepubertal girls	Fruit and vegetables, urinary calcium
Vatanparas 2005	Canada	85 boys 67 girls	Fruit and vegetables, calcium intake No association
Prynne 2006	UK	125 adolescent girls 132 adolescent boys 120 young women 70 older men 73 older women	Fruit Fruit No association No association Fruit
Chen 2006	China	670 postmenopausal women	Fruit and vegetables

In a seven-year longitudinal study of 85 boys and 67 girls aged 8-20 years, Vatanparast et al. (2005) demonstrated that, in addition to adequate dietary calcium intake, appropriate intakes of vegetables and fruit have a beneficial effect on total body bone mineral content in boys, but not in girls. In a more recent cross-sectional study, Prynne et al. (2006) explored the association between bone mineral status and fruit and vegetable intakes in 132 boys and 125 girls aged 16–18 years, in 120 young women (aged 23–37 years), and in 70 and 73 older men and women, aged 60–83 years. The authors found significant positive associations between spine size-adjusted bone mineral content and fruit intakes, in adolescent boys and girls and older women, but no significant associations were found in the young women or older men. Moreover, no significant correlation was observed between bone measurements and intake of vegetables alone (after adjustments) in any of the groups.

The association between fruit and vegetable intakes and bone health has been investigated also in intervention studies, reporting inconclusive results. In a 3 months intervention study on 23–76 years old men and women, the Dietary Approach to Stop Hypertension (the DASH diet), in which fruit and vegetable intake was increased from 3.6 to 9.5 daily servings, was associated to a significant reduction in bone turnover markers (Lin et al. 2003). More recently, Macdonald et al (2008) and McTiernan et al (2009) obtained opposite results. In the first study, 300g/day of fruit and vegetables neither influenced bone turnover, nor prevented BMD loss over 2 years in 276 healthy postmenopausal women (Macdonald et al. 2008). In the second study, in the contest of the Women's Health Initiative Dietary Modification, a low-fat and increased fruit, vegetable, and grain diet intervention did not change the risk of osteoporotic fractures in 48,835 postmenopausal women, after 8 years of follow-up.

Intervention trials in humans may help to elucidate epidemiological observations, but data are scarce as yet, and more research is needed to clarify the role of fruit and vegetables in lowering the risk of osteoporosis.

2.4. Cataract

Cataract is an important health problem that is responsible for about 30 to 50 million cases of blindness throughout the world. Cataracts increase with age, reducing visual acuity and constituting a major cause of disability in the elderly (Van Duyn & Pivonka 2000). Occurrence in the United States increases from 5% at age of 65 to 40% for persons aged 75 years and older (Taylor et al.1995). Caractogenesis is a multifactorial disease process that may be initiated or promoted by oxidative damage. Antioxidant nutrients may influence this process through their ability to scavenge free radicals and thereby reduce oxidative damage to lens tissues (Varma 1991; Taylor 1992). High plasma levels or nutrient intakes of antioxidant vitamins and long-term supplementation with vitamin C or E have been shown to be associated with diminished risk for cataracts (Jacques & Chylack 1991; Hankinson et al. 1992; Tavani et al. 1995; Olmedilla et al. 2003). From an epidemiologic point of view, the evidence of an effect of fruit and vegetables on cataract risk is limited, but promising.

The first evidence suggesting a protective role of fruits and vegetables for cataract prevention came from a case-control study by Jacques and Chylack (1991). The authors found that subjects who consumed fewer than 3.5 servings of fruit and vegetables a day had an increased risk of cataracts. In a case-control study on 1,919 participants of the Beaver Dam Eye Study, dietary folic acid, fiber, and carotenoids from vegetables were associated with a lower risk of cataracts, especially in men (Mares-Perlman et al. 1995). In a larger cohort study on 51,000 women aged 45 to 67 years, who were followed for 8 years, a high intake of dietary β-carotene and vitamin A was inversely associated with cataracts, with a 39% lower risk for higher with respect to lower consumers. Among specific food items, spinach rather than carrot (the greatest source of β-carotene) were more consistently associated with a lower risk of cataract (Hankinson et al.1992).Tavani et al. (1996) investigated the relationship between cataract incidence and diet on the basis of a case-control study conducted in northern Italy. A total of 207 patients who had cataract extraction and 706 controls were interviewed during their hospital stay. Among food items, reduced Odds Ratios (OR) for cataract was shown for higher consumption of cruciferous (OR 0.5, 95% CI 0.3-0.8), spinach (OR 0.6, 95% CI 0.4-0.9), tomatoes (OR 0.5, 95% CI 0.4-0.8), peppers (OR 0.7, 95% CI 0.4-1.1), citrus fruit (OR 0.5, 95% CI 0.2-1.3), and melon (OR 0.5, 95% CI 0.4-0.8). Spinach consumption was found to be protective against cataract also in the Nurses' Health Study. In this study, those who consumed cooked spinach ≥ 2times/week had a 30-38% lower risk of cataract than those who consumed it less than 1 times a month (Chasan-Taber et al.1999). Few years later, always in the contest of the Nurses' Health Study, Moeller et al. (2004) found that adherence to the American Dietary Guidelines, including high intakes of fruit and vegetables, was associated with a lower prevalence of age-related nuclear lens opacities in a sample of 479 participants (52 to 73 years). Decreased prevalence of nuclear opacities was observed with high intake of fruit (OR 0.58, 95% CI: 0.32-1.05) and whole grains (OR 0.64, 95% CI: 0.36-1.15). Similar results were obtained in the Health Professionals Follow-up Study. Results showed that among all the foods rich in carotenoids, broccoli and cooked spinach were inversely associated with a significantly lower risk of cataracts (Brown et al. 1999). Finally, in the Women's Health Study (WHS), with respect to lowest quintile of fruit and vegetable intake, women with higher intakes had modest, but significant 10–15% reduced risks of cataract (Christen et al. 2005).

The existing epidemiologic evidence on the association between fruit and vegetable consumption and cataract is moderately consistent with a positive effect, although more specific studies are needed in order to widely recommend an increase of fruit and vegetables for cataracts prevention.

Chapter III

Health Effects of Fruit and Vegetables: Which Mechanism of Action?

Fruit and vegetables contain a wide variety of bioactive components which can exert diverse actions *in vivo* that are potentially related to chronic disease prevention (Duthie et al. 2003; Hu, 2002; Keck & Finley, 2004). They are primary sources of dietary fiber, which comprises non-digestible polysaccharides, naturally occurring resistant starch and lignins (Panel 2001). The digestible carbohydrate component of fruit and vegetables is able to provide energy without the insurgence of sudden insulin and glycaemic peaks, while the indigestible component is able to modulate not only glycaemic response, but also blood lipids. In addition, fiber has important effects on gastrointestinal transit time. The protein component of fruit and vegetables is only minor, but contributes to regulate acid-base balance. Fruit and vegetables are basic sources of water soluble vitamins, pro-vitamin A, carotenoids and vitamin K. Folate and vitamin B6 are required to sulphuraminoacid metabolism and may contribute to decrease plasma homocystein. Fruit and vegetable are also primary potassium sources and they make a substantial contribution to maintain sodium-potassium balance, a very important mechanism to regulate blood pressure and calcium homeostasis. Plant foods are rich also in dietary antioxidants such as phenolic compounds, carotenoids and organosulfur compounds, endowed with different chemical structures and redox potentiality.

Chapter IV

Antioxidant Activity

The first action of phytochemicals is the ability to protect from the widely damaging ROS involved in several inflammatory and degenerative diseases (Halliwell & Cross 1994). Oxidative stress, which is the imbalance between ROS and antioxidant defense, can originate from an increase in free radical production either by exogenous radicals such as pollution and cigarette smoking, or by endogenous sources, such as inflammation and the respiratory burst (Davies 1995). Human antioxidant defenses have evolved to protect against ROS, and a sophisticated, co-operative array of antioxidant defense mechanisms is found in biological systems (Halliwell & Gutteridge 1989). However, despite the high grade of complexity and efficiency of the endogenous enzymatic antioxidant complex, there is a need to optimize the defense strategy against ROS with dietary antioxidants. The phytochemicals present in the human body represent an array of compounds with antioxidant activity, which are capable of coping with ROS and preventing oxidative stress.

The first evidence of the importance of antioxidants in preventing chronic diseases came from the results of the WHO/MONICA Project, showing a strong inverse correlation between plasma levels of vitamin E and ischemic heart disease (IHD) mortality, in 12 different European populations (Gey et al. 1991). On that basis, the authorsproposed the "antioxidant hypothesis", suggesting that health maintenance requires optimal internal levels of different antioxidant molecules (Gey 1986). In following years, other large prospective cohort studies investigated the association between vitamin supplementation and chronic disease prevention. Rimm et al. (1993) examined data from 39,910 US male health professionals participating to the Health Professional

Follow-up study. After checking for different variables, they found that men in the highest quintile of vitamin E intake had a significant lower relative risk of CHD (RR 0.60 ; 95% CI 0.44-0.81). The same analyses for β-carotene, showed a reduced relative risk of CHD, although this reduction resulted to be significant only in case of smoker individuals. In the Nurses' Health Study, 87,245 women aged 34 to 59 years, were followed for an average of 8 yrs (Stampfer et al. 1993). Women in the highest quintile of vitamin E intake had a 34% reduction in risk of CHD events, compared with women in the lowest quintile, but no association was recorded for β-carotene (Stampfer et al. 1993).Knekt et al. (1994) followed 2,748 men and 2,385 women aged from 30 to 69 years for 18 years. After adjusting for age and other cardiovascular risk factors, women, but not men, at the highest tertile of vitamin E intakes showed a significant reduction of CHD risk (RR 0.35, 95% CI 0.14-0.88). Vitamin C also showed significant positive effect in women (RR 0.49, 95% CI 0.24-0.98), while carotenoid intake was not correlated with a reduction in CHD risk in both men and women (Knekt et al. 1994). The Scottish Heart Health Study analyzed 4,036 men and 3,833 women from Scotland, aged 40 to 59 years, followed-up for 7.7 years. The study showed that, after adjustment for different CVD risk factors, vitamin C and β-carotene intakes were associated with a significant reduction in the incidence of new CHD events in men, but not in women, while vitamin E failed to show any positive effect (Todd et al. 1999).Finally, three large cohort studies (Rimm et al. 1993; Stampfer et al. 1993; Kushi et al. 1996), enrolling together more than 150,000 subjects did not show any association between vitamin C intake and CVD mortality.

An important contribution to the understanding of the effect of the use of antioxidant vitamins for the prevention of degenerative diseases came from randomised clinical trials, which reported either null or harmful results. In a meta-analysis of seven trials with 82,000 patients assigned to β-carotene or control group, Vivekananthan et al. (2003) showed that the rates for all-cause, cardiovascular and all-cause cerebrovascular mortality were not changed by vitamin E and slightly but significantly higher for β-carotene treatment, compared to the control group. Miller et al. (2005), in a meta-analyses including about 136,000 participants, enrolled in 19 different clinical trials, reported a statistically significant relationship between vitamin E dosage and all-cause mortality, with an increased risk for dosages higher than 150 International Unit/day. More recently, Bjelakovic et al., (2007) reviewed 68 randomized trials investigating the effect of supplementation with β-carotene, vitamin A, ascorbic acid and selenium, assumed either singly or as a combined cocktail, on all-cause mortality. Data from 232,606 participants showed that antioxidant supplementation, except for selenium and vitamin C, was able to significantly increase all-cause mortality. The results of these meta-analyses seem to raise strong concerns about the use of antioxidants for reducing cardiovascular, cerebrovascular and all-cause mortality and seem to limit their role in contributing to the protective effect of fruit and vegetables. Recent reviews of intervention human studies, reached similar conclusions (Rahaman 2007, Kamat et al. 2008, Brambilla et al. 2008, Rizzo et al 2009): although there is a relevant body of evidence supporting a causal linkage between ROS and CVD, neuro-degenerative diseases, cancer and diabetes, the evidences that treatment with antioxidants may result in a reduction of pathological effects are still scarce and difficult to interpret, seriously challenging the identification of effective antioxidant therapies.

There are some considerations worth making in order to give a clearer picture of the phenomenon. First of all, vitamin C, vitamin E and β-carotene, due to their undoubted redox properties, have gained considerable importance during the last years, becoming the centre of the redox universe. A large body of *in vitro*, in animal models and in humans' studies have furnished strong evidence of their antioxidant properties and their oxidative stress-preventing action (Benzie 2000; Evans & Halliwell 2001). However, despite this well recognized role as antioxidants, the "noble" vitamins are relatively small contributors to the overall antioxidant capacity of plant foods. The analyses of the composition of fruit and vegetables indicate the existence of hundreds of different antioxidant molecules, mostly secondary plant metabolites, such as phenolic compounds, sterols, isothiocyanatesetc, which overall, may contrib.-ute more to the fruit and vegetable redox properties (Serafini et al.1998; Serafini et al. 2000; Proteggente et al. 2002; Serafini et al. 2003;).Secondly, the concept that antioxidants "talk to each other", synergistically networking against oxidative stress, is growing (Serafiniet al. in press). Co-operation among different antioxidants provides greater protection against free radicals injury than any single compound, so that clinical trials focusing only on single molecules may well underestimate the impact of antioxidants in disease prevention. Hence, understanding the role played by antioxidant molecules in the protective effect of plant food requires more information on the overall antioxidant properties of fruit and vegetables.

The overall antioxidant properties of plant food can be assessed by measuring the Total Antioxidant Capacity (TAC), intended as the cumulative ability of food components to scavenge free radicals (Serafini & Del Rio 2004). TAC is defined as the number of moles of radicals neutralized by the tested matrix (such as food extracts or body fluids) and it is the result of many variables, such as redox potentials of the compounds present in the matrix, their cumulative and synergistic interaction, nature of the oxidizing substrate and antioxidant localization (Fig.1) (Serafini & Del Rio 2004). Recently two databases on TAC values of fruit and vegetables have been published (Halvorsen et al. 2002; Pellegrini et al. 2003).The database published by Halvorsen et al. (2002) includes data on the Ferric Reducing Antioxidant Power (FRAP), measuring the ability of the food items to donate electrons, for 32 vegetables, 23 fruits and 19 berries from different countries all around the world (cereals, nuts and pulses were also assayed).Results showed that vegetables, such as kale, chili pepper, red cabbage, parsley, artichoke, Brussels sprouts and spinach, contained higher concentrations of antioxidants, ranging from 0.98 to 2.65 mmol/100 g. The vegetables endive, cabbage, squash, fennel, cucumber and zucchini were at the bottom of the ranking, containing between 0.02 and 0.1 mmol/100g. Analyses of fruits demonstrated that pomegranates contain very high concentration of antioxidants (11.33 mmol/100g) followed by grapes, oranges, plums, pineapples, lemons, dates, kiwis, clementines and grapefruits which contained between 0.83 and 1.43 mmol/100g.Berries represented the food group with the highest antioxidant content. A TAC database of 34 vegetables, 30 fruits, 34 beverages, 6 vegetable oils, cereals, pulses, nuts, sweets and spices consumed in Italy have also been published by Pellegrini et al. (2003; 2006). TAC has been evaluated with 3 different methods in order to take account of different mechanism of action of the antioxidants: TRAP, FRAP and TEAC assays for measuring the chain-breaking antioxidant potential, the reducing power of the sample and the quenching ability in lipophilic environment, respectively.Results of the chain-breaking antioxidant potential (TRAP) of vegetables are displayed in Figure 2. The highest TAC value was found for asparagus, followed by beetroot, artichoke, turnip tops and onions. The TAC values of fruits are shown in Figure 3. Ingeneral, berries showed the highest TAC value, with blackberry being the most effective, followed by olives, plums, pineapples and oranges.

The analyses of the different DB reveal that fruit and vegetables are characterized by a large array of antioxidant potential values. This variegate redox composition of plant foods could represent a natural step contributing to the regulatory hierarchies that modulate the interaction among antioxidants in body fluids, optimizing antioxidant protection.

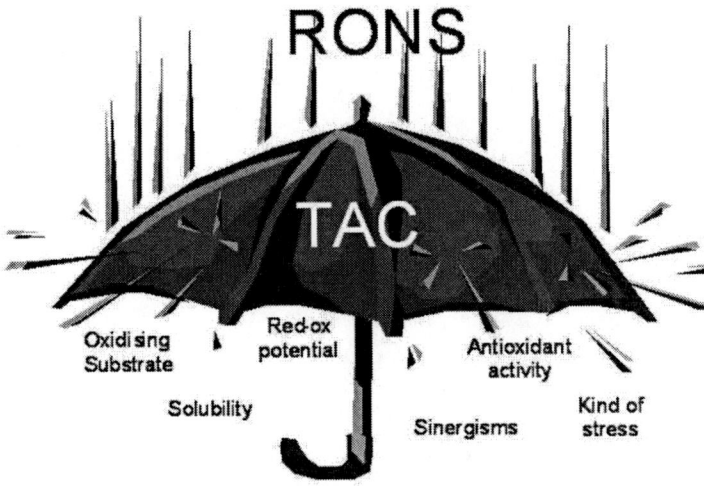

Figure 1. Variables affecting Total Antioxidant Capacity. RONS = Reactive Oxygen Nitrogen Species. Adapted from Serafini& Del Rio 2004.

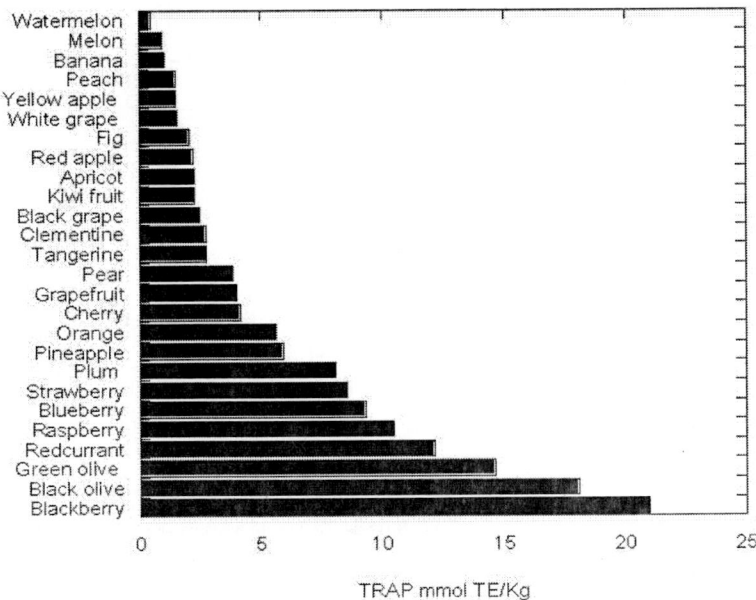

Figure 2. TAC measured as Total radical-trapping Antioxidant Potential in fruit extracts. Values are expressed as mmolTrolox/Kg of fresh weight and represent the sum of hydrophilic and lipophilic extracts. Source: Pellegrini et al. (2003).

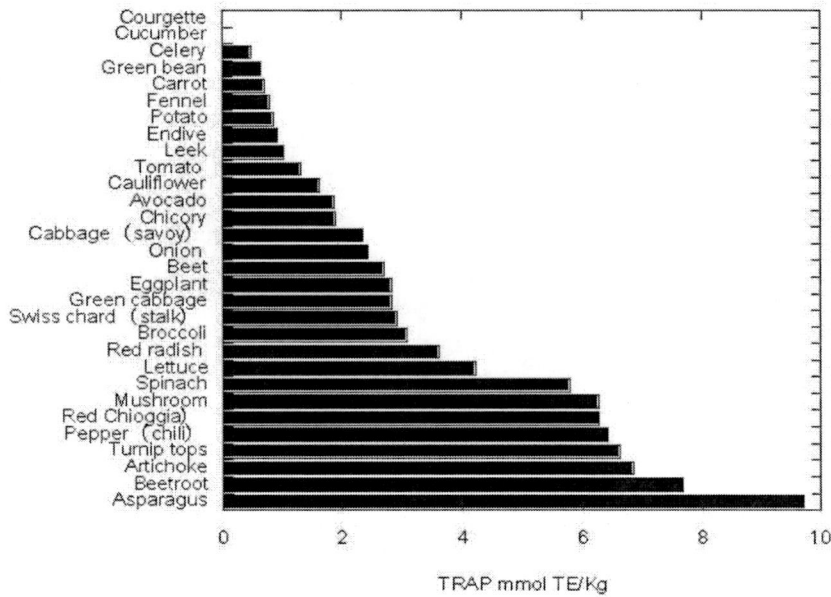

Figure 3. TAC measured as Total radical-trapping Antioxidant Potential in vegetable extracts. Values are expressed as mmolTrolox/Kg of fresh weight and represent the sum of hydrophilic and lipophilic extracts. Source: Pellegrini et al. (2003).

Despite all the speculation on the role of the redox network in preventing oxidative stress-induced diseases, its concerted impact on the incidence of pathologies has not been adequately investigated. The epidemiological application of TAC has been proposed as a tool for investigating the relationship between dietary antioxidants and gastric cancer risk in population-based case-control studies (Serafini et al. 2002).The intake of dietary TAC through plant food was inversely associated with the risk of gastric cancer, with a significant dose-response trend. Moreover, a clear dose-response relationship for increasing levels of TAC was found in smokers, while never-smokers subjects displayed a threshold effect with a similar lower risk (OR 0.48, 0.46 and 0.44) in the last 3 quartiles of intake compared to the first quartile (OR 0.56). Following the same approach Agudo et al. showed that dietary TAC from fruit and vegetables was inversely related to overall mortality rates in the Spanish cohort of EPIC.

Supplementary sources of antioxidants other than fruit and vegetables are present in the diet at very high concentration such as chocolate, tea, wine and spices. Foods, such as grain, cereals and juices, despite being endowed with a lower amount of antioxidants, may also contribute to overall antioxidant dietary intake due to their high frequency of daily consumption. In order to properly assess dietary antioxidant intake it is crucial to merge the information on dietary intake from all plant foods in an overall TAC intake, which better resembles a daily exposure to antioxidants. The potential of TAC as a descriptor of the diet, suggests that the epidemiological approach of TAC could represent a useful tool for clarifying the association between dietary antioxidants and disease.

Chapter V

Endocrine Regulation

A second core mechanism is the one that regulates gene expression through the interaction with several nuclear receptors. Among the large number of bio-active compounds present in fruit and vegetables, several are able to act through the same pathway of some hormones. Several flavonoids and lignans interact with estrogen receptors, androgen receptors, aryl receptors, thyroid receptors, modulating the action of endogenous hormones, as well as that of toxic substances.

The best known effects are the ones modulating estrogenic actions, hence the name of "phytoestrogens" given to such compounds. However, androgenic and progestinic effects should also be considered. Phytoestrogens can act as pure agonist, partial agonist or pure antagonists, according to the balance between receptor sub-types present in the different tissues and to the hormonal status. In addition, phytoestrogens may act through cell-surface (non-genomic) signalling, by regulating enzymes implicated in signal transduction, such as protein tyrosine kinase, mitogen-activated protein kinase (MAPK) and by inhibiting DNA topoisomerase II. Such effects have mainly been described for the soy phytoestrogen genistein, but several prenyl-flavonoids present in fruit and vegetables possess similar properties. Phytoestrogens are also able to modulate cell proliferation through the p38 MAPK pathway or through the phosphatidyl inositol- 3 kinase/Akt pathways. (Camper-Kirby et al., 2001; Frey & Singletary, 2003). Of all flavonoids, luteolin and naringenin display the strongest estrogenicity, while apigenin has a relatively strong progestinic activity (Zand et al. 2000). In proliferation assays using MCF-7 cells, coumestrol, daidzein, luteolin, and quercetin exerted a proliferation stimulating activity as strong as estradiol (Han et al. 2002).The endocrine regulating action can also take place by affecting hormone metabolism and bioactivity. Such action has been demonstrated in a human study in postmenopausal women that indicated that a diet rich in phytoestrogens and complex carbohydrates observed a 25 % increase of SHBG (Berrino et al. 2001).

Chapter VI

Other Mechanisms

Fibre

Dietary fiber has been associated with a reduced incidence of CVD (Pietinen et al. 1996; Rimm et al. 1996; Liu et al. 1999; Truswell 2002) and cancer (Jacobs 1988; Potter 1990; Trock et al. 1990). Potential cardiovascular benefits of dietary fiber include effects on serum lipid levels, postprandial glucose and triglyceride levels, insulin sensitivity, blood pressure (Anderson 2000; Burke et al. 2001;Panel 2002), fibrinolysis and coagulation (Pereira et al. 2000; Jenkins et al. 2000). Dietary fibre may increase fecal bulk and decrease transit time; thus, via dilution and a shorter period of contact, fiber may reduce the interaction between carcinogens and the epithelium. Moreover, certain types of fiber are fermented by microflora in the colon, leading to the production of short-chain fatty acids (Steimneitz 1996). These acids lower colonic pH and prevent from the conversion of primary to secondary bile acids, which stimulate colonic cell proliferation and are thought to promote carcinogenesis. However, despite this evidence further investigation is needed to elucidate the role of fiber in preventing chronic diseases.

Drug-Metabolizing Enzymes

Drug-metabolizing enzymes are essential for the biotransformation of endogenous compounds and in the detoxification of different xenobiotics (Yang et al. 1994). Phase I enzymes such as cytochrome P450 (CYP)-dependent monooxygenases, convert hydrophobic compounds to reactive electrophiles as a first step, before their reaction with water-soluble moieties, in order to improve excretion. Phase II enzymes, such as UDP-glucuronosyl-transferases and glutathione transferase, catalyze these conjugation reactions. Different constituents of fruit and vegetables such as flavonoids (Eaton et al. 1996), isothiocyanates (Hecht 1995) and allyl sulphides (Brady et al. 1988), have been shown to be potent modulators of CYP *in vitro* and in animal model studies. Cytochrome P450 (CYP) 3A4 appears to be especially sensitive to dietary effects, probably in relation to its high level of expression in the intestine, as well as its broad substrate specificity, but food-drug interactions involving CYP1A2, CYP2E1, glucuronosyltransferases and glutathione S-transferases have also been documented (Harris et al. 2003). However these effects are complex and are still object of debate, due to the fact that food constituents modulate CYP expression and function by a range of mechanisms, with the potential for both deleterious and beneficial outcomes (Murray 2006).

Mineral Balance

Fruit and vegetables are also a good source of potassium and magnesium. Sodium/potassium balance is a main regulator of blood pressure. Potassium is also involved in the regulation of calcium balance, and an increase in dietary potassium reduces both daily and fasting urinary calcium excretion. Magnesium is required for matrix and mineral metabolism as an essential cofactor in the function of many enzymes, including those concerned with the transfer of phosphate groups and the metabolism of ATP, but it is also required for appropriate calcium metabolism (Seelig 1993).

The Dietary Approaches to Stop Hypertension (DASH) has demonstrated that a diet rich in fruits, vegetables, low-fat dairy products, fiber and minerals (calcium, potassium and magnesium) produces a potent antihypertensive effect (Appel et al. 1997; Sacks et al., 2001).

Acid-Base Balance

The etiopatogenesis of osteoporosis has been linked to *"a life long utilisation of the buffering capacity of the basic salts of bone for the constant assault against pH homeostasis..."* Wachman & Bernstein (1968). Different dietary components have the ability to affect acid-base balance in the body.

The Potential Renal Acid Load (PRAL) is an integrated measure of such properties. Foods rich in protein such as fish, meat and certain cheeses, as well as many grains, soft beverages such as cola drinks, and most European pale beers have a high PRAL; milk and dairy products other than cheese have a low PRAL; fats and oils are neutral; and fruits, vegetables, mineral waters, coffee and wines have a negative PRAL (Remer &Manz, 1995). Typical Western diets, rich in protein from animal sources, poor in fruits and vegetables and high in salt lead to high PRAL. Mediterranean countries diets, high in fruits and vegetables, containing wine and coffee, have a lower PRAL.

Homocysteine Metabolism

A large number of case-control and prospective studies have investigated therelation of homocysteine and risk of degenerative diseases (Malinow 1999). Increased homocysteine plasma concentration (hyperhomocysteinemia) has been related to a higher risk of coronary heart disease, stroke, and peripheral vascular disease. Moreover, hyperhomocysteinemia has been postulated as a novel tumour marker (Sun et al. 2002). As much as 10% of coronary artery diseaserisk could be attributed to hyperhomocysteinemia, (Boushey et al. 1995) and a 5 µmol/L increase of plasma homocysteine has an impact on CHD risk similar to a 20 mg/dL increase inserum cholesterol. Adequate supplyof folate, vitamin B_6, vitamin B_{12}, and riboflavin from plant food reduces homocysteine levels.

Chapter VII

Conclusions

There is substantial epidemiologic and clinical evidence of a relationship between Mediterranean diet and reduced risk of all-cause mortality, CVD, cancer and other degenerative diseases (Sofi et al. 2008, Mente et al. 2009). However, the process of identifying the protective components of the diet is still controversial. In this sense, dietary flavonoids represent a class of bioactive molecules worth to be further investigated.

Based on the available data, epidemiologic evidence generally support the idea that consuming high amounts of fruit and vegetables can significantly reduce the incidence of CHD and stroke, although a causal relationship has not been demonstrated by human intervention studies, as yet. Encouraging results have been also obtained in case of cataract and osteoporosis prevention, but further research is needed. On the other hand, for what concern cancer prevention, the earlier enthusiasm coming from the promising results of case-control studieshas been hampered by latest prospective investigations and by scientific reports from panels of experts, which overall do not support the hypothesis of a solid preventive role of fruit and vegetable consumption against cancer development.

Moreover, despite both the American (USDA 2005) and European (EUFIC 2009) dietary guidelines recommend 5 or more servings of fruit and vegetables per day as a goal to achieve dietaryhealth benefits, due to the large variability in diet composition and to the difficulties of correctly calculating the population intakes of single food items, the exactrelationship between quality and quantity of fruit and vegetable intakes and diseases prevention, is far to be identified.Although investigations of dietary components are important to give insights on the mechanisms involved in dietary modulation of diseases, the emerging idea is that dietary healthy effects cannot be exclusively related to single food items, but rather to the wide array of available plant foods.

High intakes of fruits and vegetables might be also indicators of other disease-prevention life-style behaviors, including not smoking, less alcohol drinking, more exercise, less fat and calories consumption. As such, taken all together, these "healthy" practices, represent the best strategyto strengthen the defense shield against the development of degenerative diseases. Nevertheless, more clinical research is warranted in order to reveal the enormous potentiality of dietary pattern to help human being to live longer and better.

References

Agudo, A.; Cabrera, L.; Amiano, P. et al. (2007), Fruit and vegetable intakes, dietary antioxidant nutrients, and total mortality in Spanish adults: findings from the Spanish cohort of the European Prospective Investigation into Cancer and Nutrition (EPIC-Spain). *Am J Clin Nutr* 85, 1634-42.

American Heart Association. (1996), Dietary guidelines for healthy American adults. *Circulation* 94, 1795–800.

Anderson, J.W. (2000), Dietary fiber prevents carbohydrate-induced hypertriglyceridemia. *Curr. Atheroscler. Rep.* 2, 536-541.

Appel, L.J.; Moore, T.J.; Obarzanek, E. et al.(1997), A clinical trial of the effects of dietary patterns on blood pressure. DASH Collaborative Research Group. *New Engl J Med* 336, 1117-1124

Ascherio, A.; Rimm, E.B.; Hernán, M.A. et al. (1998), Intake of potassium, magnesium, calcium, and fiber and risk of stroke among US men. *Circulation* 98, 1198–1204.

Bazzano, L.A.; He, J.; Ogden, L.G. et al. (2002), Fruit and vegetable intake and risk of cardiovascular disease in US adults: the first National Health and Nutrition Examination Survey Epidemiologic Follow-up Study *Am. J. Clin. Nut.* 76, 93-99.

Benzie, J.F. (2000), Evolution of antioxidant defence mechanisms. *Eur. J. Nutr.* 39, 53-61.

Berrino, F.; Bellati, C.; Secreto, G. et al. (2001), Reducing bioavailable sex hormones through a comprehensive change in diet: the diet and androgens (DIANA) randomized trial.*Cancer Epidemiol. Biomarkers Prev.* 10, 25-33.

Bjelakovic G, Nikolova D, Gluud LL, Simonetti RG, Gluud C. (2007) Mortality in randomized trials of antioxidant supplements for primary and secondary prevention: systematic review and meta-analysis. JAMA 297, 842-57.

Block, G.; Patterson, B.; Subar, A. (1992), Fruit, vegetables, and cancer prevention: a review of the epidemiological evidence. Nutr. Cancer. 18, 1-29.

Boffetta P, Couto E, Wichmann J, Ferrari P, Trichopoulos D, Bueno-de-Mesquita HB, et al. (2010), Fruit and Vegetable Intake and Overall Cancer Risk in the European Prospective Investigation Into Cancer and Nutrition (EPIC). J Natl Cancer Inst. 102, 529-537.

Boushey, C.J.; Beresford, S.A.; Omenn, G.S. Motulsky, A.G. (1995), A quantitative assessment of plasma homocysteine as a risk factor for vascular disease. Probable benefits of increasing folic acid intakes. JAMA. 274,1049-1057.

Brady, J.F.; Li, D.C.; Ishizaki, H. Yang, C.S. (1988), Effect of diallyl sulphide on rat liver microsomal nitrosamine metabolism and other monooxygenase activities. Cancer Res. 48, 5937-5940.

Brambilla, D., Mancuso, C., Scuderi, M.R., Bosco, P., Cantarella, G., Lempereur, L., Di Benedetto, G., Pezzino, S., Bernardini, R. (2008) The role of antioxidant supplement in immune system, neoplastic, and neurodegenerative disorders: a point of view for an assessment of the risk/benefit profile. Nutrition Journal 7, 29-37.

Brown, L.; Rimm, E.B.; Seddon, J.M. et al. (1999),A prospective study of carotenoid intake and risk of cataract extraction in US men.Am. J. Clin. Nutr.70, 517-524.

Bruckdorfer K.R. (2008), Antioxidants and CVD. Proc Nutr Soc. 67, 214-22.

Burke, V.; Hodgson, J.M.; Beilin, L.J.; Giangiulioi, N.; Rogers, P. Puddley, I.B. (2001), Dietary protein and soluble fiber reduce ambulatory blood pressure in treated hypertensives. Hypertension 38, 821-826.

Camper-Kirby, D.; Welch, S.; Walker, A. et al. (2001), Myocardial Akt activation and gender: increased nuclear activity in females versus males. Circ Res.88,1020-1027.

Chasan-Taber, L.; Willett, W.C.; Seddon, J.M.et al. (1999), A prospective study of carotenoid and vitamin A intakes and risk of cataract extraction in US women.Am. J. Clin. Nutr. 70, 509-516.

Chen Yu-ming, Ho Suzanne C. and Woo Jean L.F. (2006). Greater fruit and vegetable intake is associated with increased bone mass among postmenopausal Chinese women. British Journal of Nutrition, 96, pp 745-751

Chief Medical Officer's Committee on Medical Aspects of Food and Nutrition Policy of the United Kingdom (COMA). (1998), Report of the Working Group on Diet and Cancer. Nutritional aspects of the development of cancer. Stationery Office, London.

Christen WG, Liu S, Schaumberg DA, Buring JE. (2005), Fruit and vegetable intake and the risk of cataract in women. *Am J Clin Nutr.* 81, 1417-22.

Dagenais, G.R.; Marchioli, R.; Yusuf, S. Tognoni, G. (2000), Beta-carotene, vitamin C, and vitamin E and cardiovascular diseases. *Curr. Cardiol. Rep.* 2, 293-299.

Dauchet L, Amouyel P, Dallongeville J (2009) Fruits, vegetables and coronary heart disease. *Nat Rev Cardiol.* 6: 599-608.

Dauchet L, Montaye M, Ruidavets JB, Arveiler D, Kee F, Bingham A, Ferrières J, Haas B, Evans A, Ducimetière P, Amouyel P, Dallongeville J. (2010) Association between the frequency of fruit and vegetable consumption and cardiovascular disease in male smokers and non-smokers. *Eur J Clin Nutr.* 2010, 64: 578-86.

Dauchet L., Ferrieres J., Arveiler D., Yarnell J.W., Gey F., Ducimetiere P., Ruidavets J.B., Haas B., Evans A., et al. (2004) Frequency of fruit and vegetable consumption and coronary heart disease in France and Northern Ireland: the PRIME study. *Br J Nutr* 92, 963–72.

Davies, K.J. (1995), Oxidative stress: the paradox of aerobic life. *Biochem. Soc. Symp.* 61,1-31.

De Kok T.M., van Breda M.M., Manson M.M., (2008)Mechanisms of combined action of different chemopreventive dietary compounds,*Eur J Nutr* 47: 51–59.

Diplock, A.T.; Charleaux. J-L.; Crozier-Willi, G. et al. (1998), Functional food science and defense against reactive oxidative species. *Brit. J. Nutr.* 80, S77-S112.

Doll, R. & Peto, R. (1981), *J. Natl Cancer Inst.* 66, 1191–1308.

Eaton, E.A.; Walle, U.K.; Lewis, A.J.; Hudson, T.; Wilson, A.A. Walle, T. (1996), Flavonoids, potent inhibitors of the human p-form phenolsulfotransferase. *Drug Metab. Dispos.* 24, 232-237.

Eaton-Evans, J.; McIlrath, E.M.; Jackson, W.E.; Bradley, P.; Strain, J.J. (1993), Dietary factors and vertebral bone density in perimenopausal women froma genetral medical practice in Northern Irekand. *Proc. Nutr. Soc.*52, 44A.

European Food Information Council (EUFIC) (2009). Food-based dietary guidelines in Europe. http://www.eufic.org/article/en/expid/food-based-dietary-guidelines-in-europe/

Evans, P. and Halliwell, B. (2001), Micronutrients: oxidant/antioxidant status. *Br. J. Nutr.* 85, S67-74.

Ferro-Luzzi, A. and Branca, F. (1995), Mediterranean diet, Italian-style: prototype of a healthy diet. *Am. J. Clin. Nutr.* 61,1338S-1345S.

Ferro-Luzzi, A. and Sette, S. (1989), The Mediterranean diet: an attempt to define its present and past composition. *Eur. J. Clin. Nutr.* 43, 13-29.

Feskanich, D.; Ziegler, R.G.; Michaud, D.S. et al. (2000), Prospective study of fruit and vegetable consumption and risk of lung cancer among men and women. *J. Natl. Cancer Inst.* 92,1812–23.

Frey, R.S. and Singletary, K.W. (2003), Genistein activates p38 mitogen-activated protein kinase, inactivates ERK1/ERK2 and decreases Cdc25C expression in immortalized human mammary epithelial cells. *J. Nutr.*133, 226-31.

Genkinger, J. M., Platz, e. A., Hoffman, s. C., Comstock, G. w. & Helzlsouer, K. J. (2004) Fruit, vegetable, and antioxidant intake and all-cause, cancer, and cardiovascular disease mortality in a community-dwelling population in Washington County, Maryland. *Am J Epidemiol* 160, 1223–1233.

George, S.M., Park, Y., Leitzmann, M.F., Freedman, N.D., Dowling, E.C., Reedy, J., Schatzkin, A., Hollenbeck, A., Subar A.F (2009), Fruit and vegetable intake and risk of cancer: a prospective cohort study. *Am J Clin Nutr*89, 347–53.

Gey KF, Puska P, Jordan P, Moser UK. (1991), Inverse correlation between plasma vitamin E and mortality from ischemic heart disease in cross-cultural epidemiology. Am J Clin Nutr. 53, 26S-334S.

Gey, K.F. (1986), On the antioxidant hypothesis with regard to arteriosclerosis. *Biblthca Nutr. Dieta* 37, 53-91.

Go, V.L.; Butrum, R.R. Wong, D.A. (2003), Diet, nutrition, and cancer prevention: the postgenomic era. *J. Nutr.* 133, 3830S-3836S.

Gonzalez CA, Riboli E. (2006), Diet and cancer prevention: where we are, where we are going. Nutr Cancer. 56, 225-31.

Halliwell B. Biochem J. (2007), Oxidative stress and cancer: have we moved forward? Biochem J. 401, 1-11. Halvorsen, B. L.; Holte, K., Myhrstad, et al. (2002b), A systematic screening of total antioxidants in dietary plants. *J. Nutr.* 132, 461-471.

Halliwell, B. and Cross, C.E. (1994), Oxygen-derived species: their relation to human disease and environmental stress. *Environ. Health Perspect.* 102,5-12.

Halliwell, B. and Gutteridge, J.M.C. (1989), Free radicals in biology and medicine. Clarendon Press, Oxford.

Halvorsen B.L., Holte K., Myhrstad M.C., Barikmo I., Hvattum E., Remberg S.F., et al. (2002), A systematic screening of total antioxidants in dietary plants. *J Nutr.* 132, 461-71.

Han, D.H.; Denison, M.S.; Tachibana, H. Yamada, K. (2002), Relationship between estrogen receptor-binding and estrogenic activities of environmental estrogens and suppression by flavonoids. *Biosci. Biotechnol. Biochem.* 66, 1479-1487.

Hankinson, S.E.; Stampfer, M.J.; Seddon, J.M. et al. (1992), Nutrient intake and cataract extraction in women: a prospective study.*BMJ.*305,335-339.

Harris RZ, Jang GR, Tsunoda S. (2003) Dietary effects on drug metabolism and transport, *Clin Pharmacokinet.* 42, 1071-1088.

He F.J.; Nowson C.A.; Lucas M.; MacGregor G.A. (2007), Increased consumption of fruit and vegetables is related to a reduced risk of coronary heart disease: meta-analysis of cohort studies. J Hum Hypertens. 21(9), 717-728.

He F.J.; Nowson C.A.; MacGregor G.A. (2006), Fruit an vegetable consumption and stroke: a meta-analysis of cohort studies. Lancet 367, 320-326.

Hecht, S.S. (1995), Chemoprevention by isothiocyanates. *J. Cell. Biochem.* 22, 195-209.

Heimendinger, J.; Van Duyn, M.A.; Chapelsky, D.; Foerster, S. Stables, G. (1996), The national 5 a day for better health program: a large scale nutrition intervention. *J. Public Health Manage Pract.* 2, 27-35.

Hu FB, Willett WC. (2002) Optimal diets for prevention of coronary heart disease. *JAMA*288: 2569-78.

International Agency for Research on Cancer. Fruit and Vegetables. *IARC Handbooks of Cancer Prevention* 8. Lyon, France: IARC Press; 2003.

Iuliano, L. (2001), The oxidant stress hypothesis of atherogenesis. *Lipids* 36, S41-S44.

Jacobs, L.R. (1988), Fiber and colon cancer. *Gastroenterol. Clin. North. Am.* 17,747-760.

Jacques, P.F. and Chylack, L.T. Jr. (1991), Epidemiologic evidence of a role for the antioxidant vitamins and carotenoids in cataract prevention.*Am. J. Clin. Nutr.* 53,352S-355S.

Jansen, M.C.; Bueno-de-Mesquita, H.B.; Rasanen, L. et al. (2001), Cohort analysis of fruit and vegetable consumption and lung cancer mortality in European men. *Int. J. Cancer* 92, 913–918.

Jenkins, D.J.; Axelsen, M.; Knedall, C.W.; Augustin, L.S.; Vuksan, V. Smith, U. (2000), Dietary fibre, lentecarbohydrates and the insulin-resistant diseases. *Br. J. Nutr.* 83, S157-S163.

Johnsen, S.P., Overvad, K.; Stripp, C.; Tjonneland, A.; Husted, S.E. Sorensen, H.T. (2003), Intake of fruit and vegetables and the risk of ischemic stroke in a cohort of Danish men and women*Am. J. Clin. Nutr.* 78, 57-64.

Jones, G., Riley, M.D., Whiting, S. (2001), Association between urinary potassium, urinary sodium, current diet, and bone density in prepubertal children. *Am J Clin Nutr* 73, 839–844.

Joshipura, K.J.; Ascherio, A.; Manson, J.E. et al. (1999), Fruit and vegetable intake in relation to risk of ischemic stroke. *JAMA* 282,1233–1239

Joshipura, K.J.; Hu, F.B.; Manson, J.E. et al. (2001), The effect of fruit and vegetable intake on risk for coronary heart disease. *Ann. Intern. Med.* 134,1106–1104.

Kamat CD, Gadal S, Mhatre M, Williamson KS, Pye QN, Hensley K (2008) Antioxidants in central nervous system diseases: preclinical promise and translational challenges. *J Alzheimers Dis* 15, 473–493.

Keys, A. andKeys, M. (1959) Eat well and stay well. Doubleday and Company, New York.

Knekt, P.; Jarvinen, R.; Reunanen, A.; et al. (1996),Flavonoid intake and coronary mortality in Finland: a cohort study. *Br. Med. J.* 312, 478–81.

Knekt, P.; Reunanen, A.; Jarvinen, R.; Heliovaara, M.; Maatela, J. Aromaa, A. (1994), Antioxidant vitamin intake and coronary mortality in a longitudinal population study. *Am. J. Epidemiol.* 139,1180-1189.

Kushi, L.H.; Folsom, A.R.; Prineas, R.J.; Mink, P.J.; Wu, Y. Bostick, R.M. (1996), Dietary antioxidant vitamins and death from coronary heart disease in postmenopausal women. *N. Engl. J. Med.* 334,1156–1162.

Lampe, J.W. (1999), Health effects of vegetables and fruit: assessing mechanisms of action in human experimental studies. *Am. J. Clin. Nut.* 70, 475S-490S.

Lampe, J.W. (2003), Spicing up a vegetarian diet: chemopreventive effects of phytochemicals. *Am. J. Clin. Nutr.* 78, 579S-583S.

Lanham-New SA (2006), Fruit and vegetables: the unexpected natural answer to the question of osteoporosis prevention? Am J Clin Nutr 2006;83:1254 –5.

Law, M.R. and Morris, J.K. (1998), By how much does fruit and vegetable consumption reduce the risk of ischaemic heart disease? *Eur. J. Clin. Nutr.* 52:549–556.

Lin PH, Ginty F, Appel LJ, Aickin M, Bohannon A, Garnero P, Barclay D, Svetkey LP. (2003), The DASH diet and sodium reduction improve markers of bone turnover and calcium metabolism in adults. *J Nutr.* 133, 3130-3136.

Liu, S.; Lee, I-Min,; Ajani, U.; Cole, S.R.; Buring, J.E. Manson, J.E. (2001), Intake of vegetables rich in carotenoids and risk of coronary heart disease in men: The Physicians' Health Study. *Int J Epidemiol.* 30, 130-135.

Liu, S.; Manson, J.A.E.; Lee, I-M. et al. (2000), Fruit and vegetable intake and risk of cardiovascular disease: the Women's Health Study.*Am. J. Clin. Nutr.* 72, 922-928.

Liu, S.; Stampfer, M.J.; Hu, F.B. et al.(1999), Whole grain consumption and risk of coronary heart disease: results from the nurse's health study. *Am. J. Clin. Nutr.* 70, 412-419.

Macdonald HM, Black AJ, Aucott L, Duthie G, Duthie S, Sandison R, Hardcastle AC, Lanham New SA, Fraser WD, Reid DM. (2008), Effect of potassium citrate supplementation or increased fruit and vegetable intake on bone metabolism in healthy postmenopausal women: a randomized controlled trial. *Am J Clin Nutr* 88, 465–474.

Macdonald HM, New SA, Golden MH, Campbell MK, Reid DM (2004), Nutritional associations with bone loss during the menopausal transition: evidence of a beneficial effect of calcium, alcohol, and fruit and vegetable nutrients and of a detrimental effect of fatty acids. *Am J Clin Nutr.* 79, 155-165.

Malinow, M.R. (1999), Homocysteine, vitamins and genetic interactions in vascular disease. *Can. J. Cardiol.* 15 Suppl B, 31B-34B.

Mares-Perlman, J.A.; Brady, W.E.; Klein, B.E. et al. (1995), Diet and nuclear lens opacities.*Am. J. Epidemiol.* 141,322-334.

Martínez-González, MA.; Sánchez-Villegas A. (2004), The emerging role of Mediterranean diets in cardiovascular epidemiology: monounsaturated fats, olive oil, red wine or the whole pattern? *Eur. J. Epidemiol.* 19, 9-13.

McGartland CP, Robson PJ, Murray LJ, Cran GW, Savage MJ, Watkins DC, Rooney MM, Boreham CA. (2004), Fruit and vegetable consumption and bone mineral density: the Northern Ireland Young Hearts Project. *Am J Clin Nutr.* 80, 1019-23.

McTiernan A, Wactawski-Wende J, Wu L, Rodabough RJ, Watts NB, Tylavsky F, Freeman R, Hendrix S, Jackson R; Women's Health Initiative

Investigators (2009), Low-fat, increased fruit, vegetable, and grain dietary pattern, fractures, and bone mineral density: the Women's Health Initiative Dietary Modification Trial. *Am J Clin Nutr* 89, 1864–1876.

Mente A, de Koning L, Shannon HS, Anand SS. (2009) A systematic review of the evidence supporting a causal link between dietary factors and coronary heart disease. *Arch Intern Med.* 169, 659-669.

Mente, A., De Koning, L., Shannon, H.S. & Anand, S.S. (2009) A systematic review of the evidence supporting a causal link between dietary factors and coronary heart disease. *Arch. Intern. Med.* 169, 659–669.

Michaelsson, K.; Holmberg, L.; Maumin, H.; Wolk, A.; Bergstrom, R. Ljunghall, S. (1995), Diet, bone mass and osteoclacin; a cross-sectional study. *Calc. Tissue Int.* 57, 86-93.

Michaud, D.S.; Spiegelman, D.; Clinton, S.K.; Rimm, E.B.; Willett, W.C. Giovannucci, E. (2000), Prospective study of dietary supplements, macronutrients, micronutrients, and risk of bladder cancer in US men. *Am. J. Epidemiol.* 152, 1145–1153.

Miller, E.R., Pastor-Barriuso, R., Dalal, D. et al. 2005. Meta-analysis: high dosage vitamin E supplementation may increase all-cause mortality. *Ann InternMed.* 142, 37–46.

Moeller SM, Taylor A, Tucker KL, McCullough ML, Chylack LT Jr, Hankinson SE, Willett WC, Jacques PF. (2004), Overall Adherence to the Dietary Guidelines for Americans Is Associated with Reduced Prevalence of Early Age-Related Nuclear Lens Opacities in Women. *J Nutr.* 134, 1812-9.

Murray M. (2006), Altered CYP expression and function in response to dietary factors: potential roles in disease pathogenesis. Curr Drug Metab. 7, 67-81.

Nagura, J. et al. (2009) Fruit, vegetable and bean intake and mortality from cardiovascular disease among Japanese men and women: the JACC study. *Br J Nutr.* 1–8.

Nagura, J. et al. Fruit, vegetable and bean intake and mortality from cardiovascular disease among Japanese men and women: the JACC study. Br. J. Nutr. 1–8 (2009).

Nakabeppu, Y., Tsuchimoto, D., Furuichi, M. and Sakumi, K. 2004) The defense mechanisms in mammalian cells against oxidative damage in nucleic acids and their involvement in the suppression of mutagenesis and cell death. Free Radical Res. 38, 423–429.

Nakamura, K., Nagata, C., Oba, s., Takatsuka, N., Shimizu, H. (2008) Fruit and vegetable intake andmortality from cardiovascular disease areinversely associated in Japanese women but notin men. *J Nutr* 138, 1129–1134.

Ness AR, Maynard M, Frankel S, Smith GD, Frobisher C, Leary SD, Emmett PM, Gunnell D. (2005). Diet in childhood and adult cardiovascular and all cause mortality: the Boyd Orr cohort. *Heart.* 91: 894-8.

Ness, A.R. & Powles, J.W. (1997), Fruit and vegetables, and cardiovascular disease: a review. *Int. J. Epidemiol.* 26, 1–13.

New, S.A.; Bolton-Smith, C.; Grubb, D.A. Reid, D.M. (1997), Nutritional influences on bone mineral density: a cross-sectional study in premenopausal women. *Am. J. Clin. Nutr.* 65,1831-1839.

New, S.A.; Robins. S.P.; Campbell. M.K. et al. (2000), Dietary influences on bone mass and bone metabolism: further evidence of a positive link between fuit and vegetable consumption and bone health? *Am. J. Clin. Nutr.* 71,142-151.

New, S.A.; Smith, R.; Foulds, E. Reid, D.M. (1998), Associations between present dietary intake and bone health in elderly Scottish men and women. In Current Research in Osteoporosis and Bone Mineral Measurement. Vol. 5 p.3, EFJ Ring, DM Elvins, AK Bhalla eds. London, British Institute of Radiology.

Nöthlings U, Schulze MB, Weikert C, Boeing H, van der Schouw YT, Bamia C, Benetou V, Lagiou P, Krogh V, et al. (2008) Intake of vegetables, legumes, and fruit, and risk for all-cause, cardiovascular, and cancer mortality in a European diabetic population. *J Nutr.* 138, 775-81.

Obermeier, M.T.; White, R.E. Yang, C.S. (1995), Effect of bioflavonoids on hepatic P450 activities. *Xenobiotica* 25, 575-584.

Olmedilla, B.; Granado, F.; Blanco, I. Vaquero, M. (2003), Lutein, but not alpha-tocopherol, supplementation improves visual function in patients with age-related cataracts: a 2-y double-blind, placebo-controlled pilot study.*Nutrition*19,21-24.

Panel on micronutrients, subcommittees on upper reference levels of nutrients and interpretation and uses of dietary reference intakes, and the standing committee on the scientific evaluation of dietary reference intakes, institute of medicine. Dietary reference intakes for energy, carbohydrates, fiber, fat, protein, and aminoacids (macronutrients). (2002), National Academies Press. Washington, DC.

Panel on the definition of dietary fiber, standing committee on scientific evaluation of dietary reference intakes, food and nutrition board institute of medicine. Dietary Reference Intakes: proposed definition of dietary fiber. (2001), National Academy press. Washington DC.

Parthasarathy, S.; Santanam, N. Auge, N. (1998), Oxidized low-density lipoprotein, a two faced Janus in coronary artery disease?. *Biochem. Pharmacol.* 56, 279-284.

Parthasarathy, S.; Santanam, N.; Ramachandran, S. Meilach, O. (1999), Oxidants and antioxidants in atherogenesis: an appraisal. *J. Lipid Res.* 40, 2143-2157.

Pellegrini N, Serafini M, Salvatore S, Del Rio D, Bianchi M, Brighenti F. (2006). Total antioxidant capacity of spices, dried fruits, nuts, pulses, cereals and sweets consumed in Italy assessed by three different in vitro assays. *Mol Nutr Food Res.* 50: 1030-1038.

Pellegrini, N.; Serafini, M.; Colombi, B. et al. (2003), Total antioxidant capacity of plant foods, beverages and oils consumed in Italy assessed by three different *in vitro* assays. *J. Nutr.* 133, 2812-2819.

Pereira, M.A. Pins, J.J. (2000), Dietary fiber and cardiovascular disease: experimental and epidemiologic advances. *Curr. Atheroscler. Rep.* 2, 494-502.

Pietinen, P.; Malila, N.; Virtanen, M. et al. (1999), Diet and risk of colorectal cancer in a cohort of Finnish men. *Cancer Causes Control* 10, 387–396.

Pietinen, P.; Rimm, E.B.; Korhonen, P. et al. (1996), Intake of dietary fiber and coronary heart disease in a cohort of finnish men. The alpha tocopherol, beta carotene cancer prevention study. *Circulation* 94, 2720-2727.

Potter, J.D. (1990), The epidemiology of fiber and colorectal cancer: why don't the epidemiologic data make better sense? In: Kritchevsky D Bonfield C, Anderson JW, eds Dietary fiber, New York NY Plenum Press, 431-446.

Proteggente, A. R., Pannala, A. S., Paganga, G., et al. (2002), The antioxidant activity of regularly consumed fruit and vegetables reflects their phenolic and vitamin C composition. *Free Rad. Res.* 36, 217-233.

Prynne CJ, Mishra GD, O'Connell MA, Muniz G, Laskey MA, Yan L, Prentice A, Ginty F.(2006), Fruit and vegetable intakes and bone mineral status: a cross sectional study in 5 age and sex cohorts. *Am J Clin Nutr.* 83, 1420-8.

RahmanK. (2007), Studies on free radicals, antioxidants, and co-factors. *Clinical Interventions in Aging* 2, 219–236.

Reddy, K.S. and Katan, M.B. (2004), Diet, nutrition and the prevention of hypertension and cardiovascular diseases. *Public Health Nutr.* 7, 167-186.

Reginster JY. Burlet N. Osteoporosis: A still increasing prevalence. Bone 2006;38: S4-S9

Remer, T. and Manz, F.(1995), Potential renal acid load of foods and its influence on urine pH. *J. Am. Diet. Assoc.* 95, 791-797.

Riboli. E. and Norat. T. (2003), Epidemiologic evidence of the protective effect f fruit and vegetables on cancer risk *Am. J. Clin. Nutr.* 78, 559S-569S.

Rimm, E.; Ascherio, A.; Giovannucci, E. et al. (1995), Dietary fiber intake and risk of coronary heart disease among a large population of US men. *Am. J. Epidemiol.* 141, S17 (abstr).

Rimm, E.B.; Ascherio, A.; Giovannucci, E.; Spiegelman, D.; Stampfer, M.J. Willett, W.C. (1996), Vegetable, fruit, and cereal fiber intake and risk of coronary heart disease among men. *JAMA*; 275, 447–451.

Rimm, E.B.; Stampfer, M.J.; Ascherio, A.; et al. (1993), Vitamin E consumption and the risk of coronary heart disease in men *N. Engl. J. Med.* 328,1450-1456.

Rissanen, T.H.; Voutilainen, S.; Virtanen, J.K. et al. (2003), Low intake of fruits, berries and vegetables is associated with excess mortality in men: the Kuopio Ischaemic Heart Disease Risk factor (KIHD) study. *J. Nutr.* 133,199-204.

Rizzo M., Kotur-Stevuljevic J., Berneis K., Spinas G., Rini G.B., Jelic-Ivanovic Z., Spasojevic-Kalimanovska V., Vekic J. (2009) Atherogenic dyslipidemia and oxidative stress: a new look. *Translational Research* 153, 217-223.

Ross, R. (1999), Atherosclerosis: an inflammatory disease. *N. Engl. J. Med.* 328, 1450-1456.

Royal College of Physician (2000), Osteoporosis: Clinical guidelines for prevention and treatment, London. RCP 2000.

Sacks, F.M.; Svetkey, L.P.; Vollmer, W.M. et al. (2001), DASH-Sodium Collaborative Research Group. Effects on blood pressure of reduced dietary sodium and the Dietary Approaches to Stop Hypertension (DASH) diet. DASH-Sodium Collaborative Research Group. *N. Engl. J. Med.* 344, 3-10.

Sauvaget, C. ; Nagano, J. ; Allen, N.Kodama, K. (2003), Vegetable and fruit intake and stroke mortality in the Hiroshima/Nagasaki life span study. *Stroke*, 34, 2355-2360.

Seelig, M.S. (1993) Interrelationship of magnesium and estrogen in cardiovascular and bone disorders, eclampsia, migraine and premenstrual syndrome. *J. Am. Coll. Nutr.* 12, 442-458.

Serafini M, Miglio C, Peluso I, Petrosino T. (In Press), Modulation of plasma non enzimatic antioxidant capacity (neac) by plant foods: the role of polyphenols. Current Topics in Medicinal Chemistry.

Serafini, M. and Del Rio, D. (2004), Understanding the association between dietary antioxidants, red-ox status and disease: is the Total Antioxidant Capacity the right tool?. *Redox report* 9, 145-152.

Serafini, M.; Bellocco, R.; Wolk, A. Ekström, A.M. (2002), Total Antioxidant Potential of Fruit and Vegetables and risk of gastric cancer. *Gastroenterology* 123, 985-991.

Serafini, M.; Bugianesi, R.; Maiani, M.; Valtuena, S.; De Santis, S. Crozier, A. (2003), Plasma antioxidants from chocolate. *Nature*, 424, 1013.

Serafini, M.; Laranhjinha, J.A.N.; Almeida, L. Maiani, G. (2000), Inhibition of human LDL lipid peroxidation by phenol-rich beverages and their impact on plasma Total Antioxidant Capacity (TRAP) in humans. *J. Nutr. Biochem.* 11, 585-590.

Serafini, M.; Maiani, G. Ferro-Luzzi, A. (1998), Alcohol-free red wine enhances plasma antioxidant capacity in humans. *J Nutr.* 128, 1003-1007.

Smith-Warner, S.A.; Spiegelman, D.; Yaun, S.S. et al. (2001), Intake of fruits and vegetables and risk of breast cancer: a pooled analysis of cohort studies. *JAMA* 285, 769–776.

Sofi, F. (2008), Adherence to Mediterranean diet and health status: meta-analysis. *BMJ* 337: 1344-1350.

Stampfer, M.J.; Hennekens, C.H.; Manson, J.E.; et al. (1993), Vitamin E consumption and the risk of cornary heart disease in women *N. Eng. J. Med.* 328,1444-1449.

Stary, H.C.; Chandler, A.B.; Dinsmore, R.E. et al. (1995),A definition of advanced types of atherosclerotic lesions and a histological classification of atherosclerosis. A report from the Committee on Vascular Lesions of the Council on Arteriosclerosis, American Heart Association.*Arterioscler. Thromb. Vasc. Biol.* 15,1512-1531.

Steffen LM, Jacobs Jr DR, Stevens J, Shahar E, Carithers T, Folsom AR (2003). Associations of whole-grain, refined-grain, and fruit and vegetable consumption with risks of all-cause mortality and incident coronary artery disease and ischemic stroke: the Atherosclerosis Risk in Communities (ARIC) Study. *Am J Clin Nutr* 78, 383–390.

Steinberg, D.; Witzum, J.L. (1990), Lipoproteins and atherogenesis. Current concepts. *JAMA* 264, 3047-3052.

Steinmetz, K.A. and Potter, J.D. (1996), Vegetables, fruit, and cancer prevention: a review. *J. Am. Diet. Assoc.* 96,1027–39.

Sun CF, Haven TR, Wu TL, Tsao KC, Wu JT. (2002) Serum total homocysteine increases with the rapid proliferation rate of tumor cells and decline upon cell death: a potential new tumor marker. *Clin Chim Acta.* 321, 55-62.

Surh, Y.J. (2003), Cancer chemoprevention with dietary phytochemicals. *Nat. Rev. Cancer* 3, 768-780.

Takachi, R., Inoue M., Ishihara J., Kurahashi N., Iwasaki M., Sasazuki S., Iso H, Tsubono Y., Tsugane S. (2008) Fruit and vegetable intake and risk of total cancer and cardiovascular disease: Japan Public Health Center-Based Prospective study. *Am J Epidemiol* 167, 59–70.

Tavani, A.; Negri, E. La Vecchia, C. (1996), Food and nutrient intake and risk of cataract. *Ann Epidemiol.* 6,41-46.

Tavani, A.; Negri, E.; La Vecchia, C. (1995), Selected diseases and risk of cataract in women. A case-control study from northern Italy.*Ann. Epidemiol.* 5, 234-238.

Taylor, A. (1992), Role of nutrients in delaying cataracts. *Ann. N. Y. Acad. Sci.* 669,111-23.

Taylor, A.; Jacques, P.F. Epstein, E.M. (1995), Relations among aging, antioxidant status, and cataracts. *Am. J. Clin. Nutr.* 62, 1439S-1447S.

Timothy SK, Teng S, Stolier AJ, Bolton JS, Fuhrman GM. (2002), Postmastectomy radiation in patients with four or more positive nodes.*Am Surg.* 68, 539-544

Todd, S.; Woodward, M.; Tunstall-Pedoe, H. Bolton-Smith, C. (1999), Dietary antioxidant vitamins and fiber in the aetiology of cardiovascular disease and all-cause mortality: results from the Scottish Heart Health Study. *Am. J. Epidemiol.* 150, 1073-1080.

Trichopoulou A., Bamia C., Trichopoulos D. (2009) Anatomy of health effects of Mediterranean diet: Greek EPIC prospective cohort study. *BMJ.*23, 338.

Trock, B.; Lanza, E. Grennwald, P. (1990), Dietary fiber, vegetables, and colon cancer: critical review and meta-analyses of the epidemiologic evidence. *J. Natl. Cancer Inst.* 82, 650-661.

Truswell, A.S. (2002), Cereal grains and coronary heart disease. *Eur. J. Clin. Nutr.* 56, 1-14.

Tucker, K.L.; Hannan, M.T.; Chen, H.; Cupples, A.; Wilson, P.W.F. Kiel, D.P. (1999), Potassium and fruit and vegetables are associated with greater bone mineral density in elderly men and women. *Am.J. Clin. Nutr.* 69, 727-736.

Tylavsky FA. (2004), Nutrition influences bone growth in children. *J Nutr* 134, 689S-690S.

U.S. Department of Health and Human Services and U.S. Department of Agriculture (2005), Dietary Guidelines for Americans, 2005. 6th Edition, Washington, DC: U.S. Government Printing Office.

US Department of Agriculture, US Department of Health and Human Services. (1995), Nutrition and your health: dietary guidelines for Americans. Washington, DC: US Government Printing Office.

Van Duyn, M.A. and Pivonka, E. (2000), Overview of the health benefits of fruit and vegetable consumption for the dietetics professional: selected literature *J. Am. Diet. Assoc.* 100, 1511-1521.

Van't Veer, P.; Jansen, M.C.J.F.; Klerk, M. Kok, FJ. (2000), Fruits and vegetables in the prevention of cancer and cardiovascular disease. *Public Health Nutr*.3,103–107.

Varma, SD. (1991), Scientific basis for medical therapy of cataracts by antioxidants. *Am. J. Clin. Nutr.* 53, 335S-345S;

Vatanparast H, Baxter-Jones A, Faulkner RA, Bailey DA, Whiting SJ. (2005), Positive effects of vegetable and fruit consumption and calcium intake on bone mineral accrual in boys during growth from childhood to adolescence: the University of Saskatchewan Pediatric Bone Mineral Accrual Study. *Am J Clin Nutr.* 82, 700-6.

Vivekananthan, D.P.; Penn, M.S.; Sapp, S.K.; Hsu, A. Topol, E.J. (2003), Use of antioxidant vitamins for the prevention of cardiovascular disease: meta-analysis of randomized trials *Lancet*; 361, 2017-2023.

Voorrips, L.E.; Goldbohm, R.A.; Verhoeven, D.T. et al. (2000), Vegetable and fruit consumption and lung cancer risk in the Netherlands Cohort Study on diet and cancer. *Cancer Causes Control* 11, 101–115.

Wachman, A. and Bernstein, D.S. (1968), Diet and osteoporosis.*Lancet* 7549, 958-959.

Whiting, S.J.; Boyle, J.L.; Thompson, A.; Mirwald, R.L. Faulkner, R.A. (2002), Dietary protein, phosphorus and potassium are beneficial to bone mineral density in adult men consuming adequate dietary calcium. *J. Am. Coll. Nutr.* 5, 402-409.

WHO/FAO Expert consultation on diet, nutrition and the prevention of chronic diseases. (2003), Diet, nutrition and the prevention of chronic diseases report of ajoint WHO/FAO expert consultation. *WHO Technical report series*, 916, Geneva, Switzerland.

Witzum, J.L. and Steinberg, D. (2001), The oxidative modification hypothesis of atherosclerosis: does it hold for humans? Trends *Cardiovasc. Med.* 11,93-102.

World Cancer Research Fund. (1997) Food, nutrition and the prevention of cancer: a global perspective. Washington, DC: American Institute for Cancer Research.

World Cancer Research Fund/American Institute for Cancer Research. Food, Nutrition, Physical Activity and the Prevention of Cancer: A Global Perspective. Washington, DC: AICR; 2007.

Yang, C.S.; Smith, T.J. Hong, J-Y. (1994), Cytochrome P-450 enzymes as targets for chemoprevention against chemical carcinogenesis and toxicity: opportunities and limitations. *Cancer Res.* 54, 1982S-1986S.

Zand, R.S.; Jenkins, D.J. Diamandis E.P. (2000) Steroid hormone activity of flavonoids and related compounds. *Breast Cancer Res. Treat.* 62, 35-49.

Index

A

acid, 1, 23, 37, 51
activity level, 18
adjustment, 6, 12, 18, 26
adolescent boys, 19, 20
aetiology, 53
agonist, 33
alcohol consumption, 6
alpha-tocopherol, 49
Alzheimer's diseases, 1
American Heart Association, 41, 52
androgen, 33
androgens, 41
antioxidant, 2, 20, 25, 26, 27, 28, 31, 41, 42, 44, 45, 46, 50, 52, 53, 54
arteries, 10, 11
arteriosclerosis, 44
artery, 11
ascorbic acid, 26
Asia, 13
assault, 37
assessment, 42
atherogenesis, 45, 50, 53
atherosclerosis, 11, 52, 55
ATP, 36
authorities, 10

B

behaviors, 40
beneficial effect, 19, 47
beverages, 28, 37, 50, 52
bile, 35
bile acids, 35
bioactive non-nutrient compounds, i, 2
Biochemical, 1
bioflavonoids, 49
biological systems, 25
biomarkers, 18
blindness, 20
blood pressure, 23, 35, 36, 41, 42, 51
blood vessels, 10
body fluid, 27, 28
body weight, 18
Boeing, 49
bone, 17-20, 36, 42, 43, 46-50, 52, 54
bone growth, 54
bone mass, 17, 18, 42, 48, 49
bone mineral content, 19
breast cancer, 9, 52
Britain, 13

C

cabbage, 28

calcification, 11
calcium, 9, 17, 18, 19, 23, 36, 41, 47, 54
campaigns, 2
cancer, vii, 2, 5, 6, 7, 8, 9, 10, 27, 30, 35, 39, 42, 43, 44, 48-55
cancer cells, 5
cancer prevention, vii, 39, 42, 44, 50, 53
carbohydrate, 23, 41
carbohydrates, 1, 49
carcinogen, 5
carcinogenesis, 5, 6, 35, 55
Carcinogenesis, 5
cardiovascular disease (CVD), 1, 13, 41, 43, 44, 47, 48, 49, 50, 51, 53, 54
cardiovascular risk, 12, 26
cardiovascular system, 11
carotene, 21, 26, 27, 43, 50
carotenoids, 21, 23, 45, 47
cataract, 21, 22, 39, 42, 43, 45, 53
cataract extraction, 21, 42, 45
causal relationship, 39
cell death, 49, 53
central nervous system, 46
cerebrovascular, 26
cervix, 6, 7
chain-breaking antioxidant potential (TRAP), 28
cheese, 37
chemical structures, 2, 23
chemoprevention, 53, 55
Chief Medical Officer's Committee on Medical Aspects of Food and Nutrition Policy of the United Kingdom (COMA), 7
childhood, 13, 18, 49, 54
China, 19
Chinese women, 18, 43
cholesterol, 2, 37
chronic diseases, 25, 35, 55
cigarette smoking, 25
class, 10, 39
climate, 1
clinical, 1, 11, 17, 26, 27, 39, 40, 41
clinical trials, 26, 27
clonal proliferation, 5

coffee, 37
colon, 6, 7, 9, 35, 45, 53
colon cancer, 45, 53
color, iv
colorectal cancer, 50
community, 44
complement, 5
complex carbohydrates, 34
complexity, 25
composition, 27, 28, 44, 50
compounds, vii, 1, 2, 23, 25, 27, 28, 33, 35, 43, 55
confounders, 6, 17
confounding variables, 10
conjugation, 36
consensus, 1, 2
consumption, vii, 1, 2, 3, 6, 7, 8, 11, 12, 17, 18, 21, 22, 31, 39, 40, 43-49, 51, 52, 54
control group, 26
controlled trials, 17
copyright, iv
coronary artery disease, 37, 50, 52
coronary heart disease, 11, 37, 43, 45, 46, 47, 48, 50, 51, 53
correlation, 18, 20, 25, 44
correlations, 17, 19
cross-sectional study, 18, 19, 48, 49
culture, 2
CVD, 1, 10, 11, 12, 14, 15, 17, 26, 27, 35, 39, 42
cytochrome, 35
cytokines, 11

D

damages, iv
database, 28
deaths, 12, 13
defence, 41
defense mechanisms, 25, 48
degenerative diseases, vii, 25, 26, 37, 39, 40
Denmark, 14
Department of Agriculture, 54
Department of Health and Human Services, 54

detoxification, 2, 35
diabetes, 12, 27
diagnosis, 17
diet, vii, 1, 2, 6, 8, 9, 12, 17, 20, 21, 30, 34, 36, 39, 41, 44, 46, 47, 51, 52, 53, 54, 55
diet composition, 39
dietary fiber, 23, 35, 50
dietary intake, 8, 9, 31, 49
disability, 20
DNA, 6, 33
DNA damage, 6
dosage, 26, 48
dose-response relationship, 30
drug interaction, 36
drug metabolism, 45
dyslipidemia, 51

E

electrons, 28
endocrine, 33
environmental change, 2
environmental factors, 5, 6
enzymes, 2, 6, 33, 35, 36, 55
epidemiologic studies, 12
epidemiological research, 1
epidemiology, 44, 47, 50
epigenetic modulations, 5
epithelial cells, 44
epithelium, 35
esophagus, 6, 7, 9
estrogen, 33, 45, 52
European Prospective Investigation into Cancer and Nutrition (EPIC), 13
excretion, 18, 36
exercise, 40
experimental evidence, 2
exposure, 31

F

fasting, 36
fat, 1, 20, 36, 40, 48, 49

fatty acids, 35, 47
fiber, 18, 19, 21, 23, 35, 36, 41, 42, 49, 50, 51, 53
fibrinolysis, 35
Finland, 14, 46
fish, 1, 37
flavonoids, 33, 36, 39, 45, 55
folate, 12, 37
folic acid, 21, 42
food intake, 18
fractures, 20, 48
fragility, 17
France, 14, 15, 43, 45
free radicals, 20, 27, 50
fruits, 2, 6, 8, 10, 12, 13, 18, 21, 28, 36, 37, 40, 50, 51, 52

G

gene amplification, 6
gene expression, 5, 33
genetic alteration, 5
geography, 1
glucose, 35
glutathione, 36
growth factor, 11
guidelines, 2, 39, 41, 44, 51, 54

H

health effects, 53
health status, 52
heart disease, 2, 25, 44, 52
height, 18
hemorrhage, 11
homeostasis, 23, 37
homocysteine, 37, 42, 53
hypertension, 12, 51
hypertriglyceridemia, 41
hypothesis, 25, 39, 44, 45, 55

I

immune function, 2

immune system, 42
in vivo, 6, 23
incidence, 1, 6, 8, 10, 13, 14, 17, 21, 26, 30, 35, 39
inflammation, 6, 25
inflammatory disease, 51
initiation, 5
inositol, 33
insulin, 23, 35, 46
insulin sensitivity, 35
intervention, 8, 12, 17, 20, 27, 39, 45
intestine, 36
ionizing radiation, 5
Ireland, 14, 15
iron, 1, 9
ischaemic heart disease, 47
ischemic heart disease (IHD), 25
Italy, 21, 28, 50, 53

J

Japan, 12, 14, 15, 53
Japanese women, 49
Jordan, 44

K

kidney, 7

L

larynx, 6, 7, 8, 9
LDL, 11, 52
lens, 20, 21, 47
lesions, 11, 52
lignans, 33
lipid peroxidation, 11, 52
lipids, 11, 23
lipoproteins, 11
liver, 7, 10, 42
localization, 28
longitudinal study, 18, 19
low-density lipoprotein, 50
lung cancer, 9, 44, 46, 54

M

macronutrients, 48, 49
macrophages, 11
magnesium, 9, 17, 18, 19, 36, 41, 52
markers, 17, 20, 47
matrix, 27, 36
meat, 1, 37
Mediterranean, vii, 1, 17, 37, 39, 44, 47, 52, 53
Mediterranean countries, 37
melon, 21
menopause, 18
meta-analysis, 9, 12, 26, 42, 45, 52, 54
metabolism, 2, 23, 34, 36, 42, 47, 49
metabolites, 27
metabolizing, 35
micronutrients, 48, 49
mineral water, 37
mitogen, 33, 44
mitogen activated protein kinase (MAPK), 33
modification, 55
molecules, 2, 6, 25, 27, 39
monounsaturated fatty acids, 17
mortality rate, 30
mutagen, 5
mutagenesis, 49
mutated cells, 5
mutation, 5

N

National Institutes of Health, 10
necrosis, 11
Netherlands, 54
networking, 27
neurodegenerative disorders, 42
nodes, 53
non-smokers, 43
North America, 12
Northern Ireland, 19, 43, 48
nuclear receptors, 33
nucleic acid, 49

Index

nutrients, 5, 11, 17, 20, 41, 47, 49, 53
nutrition, 7, 44, 45, 50, 51, 55

O

olive oil, 1, 47
opportunities, 55
oral cavity, 6
organ, 5
osteoporosis, 17, 20, 36, 39, 46, 54
oxidation, 11
oxidative damage, 20, 48
oxidative stress, 6, 11, 25, 27, 30, 51

P

pancreas, 6, 7, 10
Parkinson's, 1
pathogenesis, 48
pathways, 33
peripheral vascular disease, 37
permission, iv
peroxidation, 11
pharynx, 7, 8, 9
phenol, 52
phosphorus, 9, 54
photoprotectants, 2
physical activity, 10
phytochemicals, vii, 2, 25, 46, 53
pilot study, 49
placebo, 49
plant food-based diets., vii
Plant-based foods, vii, 1
plants, 44, 45
plaque, 11
plasma levels, 20, 25
platelet aggregation, 2
point mutation, 6
pollution, 25
polyphenols, 52
positive correlation, 18
postmenopausal women, 17, 19, 20, 34, 46, 47
potassium, 1, 9, 17-19, 23, 36, 41, 46-47, 54

premenstrual syndrome, 52
prevention, vii, 2, 9, 11, 17, 21, 22, 23, 25, 26, 27, 39, 40, 42, 44-46, 50, 51, 53-55
pro-atherogenic, 11
proliferation, 5, 33, 35, 53
protective role, vii, 9, 17, 21
prototype, 44
public awareness, 2
public health, 2

Q

quartile, 30

R

radiation, 53
radicals, 25, 27, 45
radius, 18
reactions, 36
Reactive Oxygen Nitrogen Species (RONS), 6
recall, 8
receptors, 33
recommendations, iv, 7
rectum, 6, 7, 8, 9
riboflavin, 37
rights, iv
risk factors, 12, 17, 26

S

salts, 36
saturated fat, 1
saturated fatty acids, 1
screening, 44, 45
selenium, 26
serum, 35
sex, 6, 41, 50
sex hormones, 41
signal transduction, 33
signalling, 33
smoking, 6, 18, 40
smooth muscle, 11

smooth muscle cells, 11
social class, 18
sodium, 9, 23, 46, 47, 51
soy phytoestrogen genistein, 33
Spain, 41
species, 11, 43, 45
speculation, 30
spine, 19
starch, 1, 23
sterols, 27
stomach, 6, 7, 9
stroke, 11-14, 37, 39, 41, 45, 46, 51, 52
sulphur, 23
Sun, 37, 53
suppression, 45, 49
susceptibility, 17
Sweden, 19
Switzerland, 55

T

therapy, 54
thrombosis, 11
thyroid, 7, 33
tissue, 17
Total Antioxidant Capacity (TAC), 27
toxic substances, 33
toxicity, 55
transport, 45
trial, 41, 47
tumor, 5, 6, 53
tumor cells, 53
tumor growth, 5
tumorigenesis, 6
turnover, 17, 20, 47
tyrosine, 33

U

United Kingdom, 7, 8, 43
United Nations, 12
universe, 27

urine, 51
US Department of Health and Human Services, 54
USDA, 2, 39

V

vegetable kingdom, vii
vegetable oil, vii, 28
vegetables, vii, 1, 2, 3, 6-12, 14, 17-23, 27, 28, 30, 33, 36, 37, 39, 40, 42, 43, 45, 46, 47, 49-54
visual acuity, 20
vitamin A, 21, 23, 26, 42
vitamin B1, 37
vitamin B12, 37
vitamin B6, 23, 37
vitamin C, 17, 18, 19, 20, 26, 27, 43, 50
vitamin D, 1
vitamin E, 25, 26, 27, 43, 44, 48
vitamin K, 23
vitamin supplementation, 25
vitamins, 1, 9, 20, 23, 26, 27, 45-47, 53, 54

W

wealth, 2
World Cancer Research Fund with the American Institute for Cancer Research (WCRF-AICR), 7
World Health Organisation, 12

Y

young women, 19

Z

zinc, 1